Atlas of Pathological Computer Tomography
Volume 3

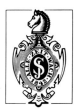

L. Jeanmart   A. L. Baert   A. Wackenheim

Computer Tomography of Neck, Chest, Spine, and Limbs

With the Collaboration of M. Osteaux

With Contributions by

D. Baleriaux, M. Bard, P. Biondetti, J. A. Bulcke,
T. Darras, D. De Becker, P. De Maeyer, P. De Somer,
L. Divano, W. Döhring, J. Ferrané, W.A. Fuchs,
A. Grivegnée, H. Hauser, N. Hermanus, D. Larde,
M. Lemort, C. Massare, M. Nijssens, M. Osteaux,
S. Sintzoff, T. Stadnik, M. Stienon, L. Ticket,
N. Vasile, P. Vock, S. Vukanovic

With 545 Figures

Springer-Verlag
Berlin Heidelberg New York Tokyo 1983

ISBN 3-540-11439-4 Springer-Verlag Berlin Heidelberg New York Tokyo
ISBN 0-387-11439-4 Springer-Verlag New York Heidelberg Berlin Tokyo

Library of Congress Cataloging in Publication Data. Jeanmart, L., 1929– Computer tomography of neck, chest, spine, and limbs. (Atlas of pathological computer tomography; v. 3) Bibliography: p. Includes index. 1. Chest—Radiography—Addresses, essays, lectures. 2. Neck—Radiography—Addresses, essays, lectures. 3. Spine—Radiography—Addresses, essays, lectures. 4. Extremities (Anatomy)—Radiography—Addresses, essays, lectures. 5. Tomography—Addresses, essays, lectures. I. Baert, A.L., 1931–. II. Wackenheim, A. (Auguste), 1925–. III. Title. IV. Series. [DNLM: 1. Abdomen—Radiography. 2. Brain—Radiography—Atlases. 3. Skull—Radiography—Atlases. 4. Tomography, X-ray computed—Atlases. WN 17 W115a 1980]. RC941.J4 1983 616.07′572 83-4655 ISBN 0-387-11439-4 (U.S.)

Reproduction of the figures: Gustav Dreher GmbH, Stuttgart
Typesetting, printing and bookbinding: Universitätsdruckerei H. Stürtz AG, Würzburg
2121/3130-543210

Authors and Collaborators

Jeanmart, Louis, Professor and Chairman of Department of Diagnostic Radiology, Institut Jules Bordet, Rue Heger Bordet, 1, B-1000 Bruxelles

Baert, Albert L., Professor and Chairman of Department of Diagnostic Radiology, Universitaire Ziekenhuizen, Capucijnenvoer, 35, B-3000 Leuven

Wackenheim, Auguste, Professor and Chairman of Department of Diagnostic Radiology, CHU Strasbourg, 1, Place de l'Hôpital, F-67005 Strasbourg Cedex

Osteaux, M., Professeur Agrégé, Department of Radiology, Institut Jules Bordet, Université Libre, Rue Heger Bordet, 1, B-1000 Bruxelles

Baleriaux, D., Senior Staff Member of Department of Radiology, Hôpital Erasme, Route de Lennik, 808, B-1070 Bruxelles

Bard, M., Radiologiste des Hôpitaux de Paris, Scanner Interclinique Hartman (Neuilly-Paris), Rue Alfred Bruneau, 5, F-75016 Paris

Biondetti, P., Resident of Department of Radiology, Instituto di Radiologia Via Giustimani, 2, I-35100 Padova

Bulcke, J.A., Senior Staff Member of Department of Neurology and Neurosurgery, A.Z. St. Rafael, K.U.B., Capucijnenvoer, 35, B-3000 Leuven

Darras, T., Senior Staff Member, Department of Radiology, Hôpital Civil de Charleroi, B-6000 Charleroi

De Becker, D., Resident of Department of Radiology, Institut Jules Bordet, Rue Heger Bordet, 1, B-1000 Bruxelles

De Maeyer, P., Resident of Department of Radiology, A.Z. St. Rafael, K.U.B., Capucijnenvoer, 35, B-3000 Leuven

De Somer, P., Resident of Department of Radiology, A.Z. St. Rafael, K.U.B., Capucijnenvoer, 35, B-3000 Leuven

Divano, L., Resident of Department of Radiology, Institut Jules Bordet, Rue Heger Bordet, 1, B-1000 Bruxelles

Döhring, W., Abteilung Diagnostische Radiologie I der Medizinischen Hochschule Hannover, Konstanty-Gutschow-Straße 8, D-3000 Hannover 61

Ferrané, J., Professor and Chairman of Department of Radiology, Hôpital Henri Mondor, 51, Avenue du Maréchal de Lattre de Tassigny, F-94010 Creteil

Fuchs, W.A., Professor and Chairman of Institute of Diagnostic Radiology, University of Bern, Inselspital Bern, CH-3010 Bern

Grivegnée, A., Resident of Department of Radiology, Hôpital Saint-Pierre, Rue Haute, 322, B-1000 Bruxelles

Hauser, H., Senior Staff Member of Institut Universitaire de Radiologie, Hôpital Cantonal, CH-1211 Geneve

Hermanus, N., Resident of Department of Radiology, Hôpital Brugmann, Place Van Gehuchten, 4, B-1020 Bruxelles

Larde, D., Senior Staff Member of Department of Radiology, Hôpital Henri Mondor, 51, Avenue du Maréchal de Lattre de Tassigny, F-94010 Creteil

Lemort, M., Resident of Department of Radiology, Institut Jules Bordet, Rue Heger Bordet, 1, B-1000 Bruxelles

Massare, C., Attaché de Consultation de Radiologie des Hôpitaux de Paris, Scanner Interclinique Hartman (Neuilly-Paris), 5, Rue Alfred Bruneau, F-75016 Paris

Nijssens, M., Resident of Department of Radiology, A.Z. St. Rafael, K.U.B., Capucijnenvoer, 35, B-3000 Leuven

Sintzoff, S., Chairman of Department of Radiology, Clinique du Parc Léopold, Rue Froissart, 38, B-1040 Bruxelles

Stadnik, T., Resident of Department of Radiology, Institut Jules Bordet, Rue Heger Bordet, 1, B-1000 Bruxelles

Stienon, M., Resident of Department of Radiology, Institut Jules Bordet, Rue Heger Bordet, 1, B-1000 Bruxelles

Ticket, L., Resident of Department of Radiology, Hôpital Brugmann, Place Van Gehuchten, 4, B-1020 Bruxelles

Vasile, N., Professeur Agrégé, Department of Radiology, Hôpital Henri Mondor, 51, Avenue du Maréchal de Lattre de Tassigny, F-94010 Creteil

Vock, P., Senior Staff Member of Institute of Diagnostic Radiology, University of Bern, Inselspital Bern, CH-3010 Bern

Vukanovic, S., Senior Staff Member of Institut Universitaire de Radiologie, Hôpital Cantonal, CH-1211 Geneve

Preface

The purpose of this book is to provide the radiologist with information which is "as practical as possible" for the everyday use of computerized tomography (CT) in the field of cervical, thoracic, and musculoskeletal pathology.

The approach is simple. For each region the following information is presented: (1) a general schematic introduction, summarizing the main indications for CT and its specific usefulness; (2) a series of pictures of normal structures with a precise and practical identification; and (3) a selection of pictures of pathological structures, with a description and a short comment, aimed at covering the largest possible field of CT indications and interests.

This approach has been applied to the following areas: cervical pathology, with one section dealing with the larynx and hypopharynx; the thorax, specifically to pulmonary diseases, pleural and parietal pathology, and the mediastinum, with special sections dealing with tumours, the heart, and large vessels; the spine, which is of growing importance in clinical CT; and finally the pathology of the musculoskeletal system in general, with special attention being paid to the developing field of orthopaedic CT measuring methods.

As the subjects covered are many and diverse, and since a broad sample of pathological cases was required, a large and geographically widespread group of specialists in specific fields were asked to collaborate. We would like to thank all of the contributors for their efforts and cooperation during the preparation of this work. We would also like to extend special thanks to Dr. A. GRIVEGNÉE for his help in reviewing the material.

Finally, we are very grateful to the staff of Springer-Verlag, Heidelberg, for their competence and patience in the difficult task of dealing with material of such diverse origins.

L. JEANMART A. BAERT A. WACKENHEIM and M. OSTEAUX

Contents

Chapter 4 Mediastinum

A.L. BAERT, P. BIONDETTI, T. DARRAS, P. DE SOMER, L. DIVANO,
J. FERRANÉ, A. GRIVEGNÉE, H. HAUSER, L. JEANMART, D. LARDE,
M. NIJSSENS, M. OSTEAUX, and N. VASILE

Chapter 5 Spine

D. BALERIAUX, L. DIVANO, N. HERMANUS, M. LEMORT, M. STIENON,
and L. TICKET

Chapter 6 Musculoskeletal System: Girdles and Limbs

M. BARD, C. MASSARE, and S. SINTZOFF

Chapter 7 Myopathies

J.A. Bulcke and P. De Maeyer. Figs. 7.1–7.5

CHAPTER 1

Neck

D. De Becker, M. Osteaux, T. Stadnik, M. Stienon, and S. Vukanovic

1.1 Technique and Normal Anatomy

T. Stadnik, D. De Becker, M. Stienon, and M. Osteaux

Fast scanning and good spatial resolution are both essential to obtain a good morphological representation of the neck. Indeed, the motility of pharyngolaryngeal structures necessitates a short scanning time. The narrowness of the fatty spaces and the small differences in density between muscles, vessels and nerves demand high spatial and densitometric resolution.

The following images were realized with a third-generation scanner. Scan time is 5 s, and slice thickness is 2 mm in order to decrease the partial volume effect. The patient lies supine with the neck in extension to obtain transverse sections of laryngeal structures. The head is fixed. Laryngeal examinations are performed with the patient breathing lightly. Phonation scans can be obtained in order to study vocal cord motility. Other neck structures are visualized in apnoea. If necessary, vessels are studied after fast i.v. injection of contrast media or with i.v. perfusion.

Fig. 1.1. Hyoid bone level (C4). The two internal jugular veins are frequently of different sizes, but this often has no pathological significance. The epiglottis is seen as a thin lamella. In front of it are the valleculae, which are symmetrical in this case but are frequently asymmetrical.

1 C4 body
2 Articular process
3 Hyoid bone body
4 Greater horn of hyoid bone
5 Medial glosso-epiglottic fold
6 Pharyngolaryngeal fold
7 Epiglottis
8 Vallecula
9 Platysma muscle
10 Digastric muscle tendinous insertion
11 Sternocleidomastoid muscle
12 Longus cervicis muscle
13 Semispinalis cervicis muscle, multifidus muscle, rotator muscle
14 Semispinalis capitis muscle
15 Longissimus capitis muscle
16 Splenius muscle
17 Levator scapulae muscle
18 Trapezius muscle
19 Submandibular gland
20 Internal carotid artery
21 External carotid artery
22 Internal jugular vein
23 External jugular vein
24 Anterior jugular vein
25 Vertebral artery

Fig. 1.2. C6 level. The narrowness of laryngeal lumen is due to apnoea. The common carotid artery is still seen on the left. On the right, the common carotid artery has divided into the internal and external carotid arteries. The vertebral arteries are seen in the transverse foramina.

1 C6 body
2 Articular process
3 Vertebral lamina
4 Thyroid cartilage
5 Arytenoid cartilage
6 Ventricular fold
7 Laryngeal ventricle
8 Sternothyroid muscle, sternohyoid muscle
9 Sternocleidomastoid muscle
10 Longus cervicis muscle
11 Inferior constrictor muscle of pharynx
12 Multifidus muscle, rotator muscle
13 Semispinalis cervicis muscle
14 Splenius muscle
15 Levator scapulae muscle
16 Trapezius muscle
17 Scalenus medius and posterior muscles
18 Scalenus anterior muscle
19 Common carotid artery
20 Internal jugular vein
21 Internal carotid artery
22 External carotid artery
23 Superior thyroid artery
24 External jugular vein
25 Anterior jugular vein
26 Vertebral artery

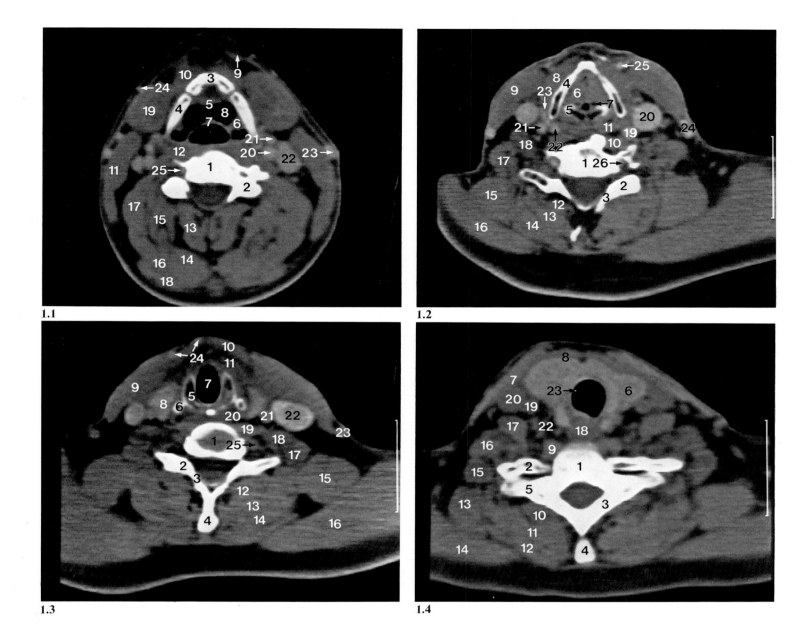

Fig. 1.3. C7 level. The lateral lobe of the thyroid gland can be seen. The vertebral artery has not yet entered the transverse foramen of the cervical vertebra.

1 C7 body	*14* Splenius muscle
2 Articular process	*15* Levator scapulae muscle
3 Vertebral lamina	*16* Trapezius muscle
4 Spinous process	*17* Scalenus medius and posterior
5 Cricoid cartilage	muscles
6 Inferior horn of thyroid	*18* Scalenus anterior muscle
cartilage	*19* Longus cervicis muscle
7 Trachea	*20* Inferior constrictor muscle of
8 Thyroid gland	pharynx
9 Sternocleidomastoid muscle	*21* Common carotid artery
10 Sternocleidohyoid muscle	*22* Internal jugular vein
11 Sternothyroid muscle	*23* External jugular vein
12 Multifidus muscle	*24* Anterior jugular vein
13 Complexus muscle	*25* Vertebral artery

Fig. 1.4. D1 level. The section passes through the thyroid gland isthmus. The high density of the thyroid gland is due to its high iodine content.

1 D1 body	*12* Splenius muscle
2 First rib	*13* Levator scapulae muscle
3 Vertebral lamina	*14* Trapezius muscle
4 Spinous process	*15* Scalenus posterior muscle
5 Transverse process	*16* Scalenus medius muscle
6 Thyroid gland	*17* Scalenus anterior muscle
7 Sternocleidomastoid	*18* Oesophagus
muscle	*19* Common carotid artery
8 Sternohyoid muscle,	*20* Internal jugular vein
sternothyroid muscle	*21* External jugular vein
9 Longus cervicis muscle	*22* Vertebral artery, inferior
10 Multifidus muscle	thyroid artery, nerve trunks
11 Complexus muscle	*23* Trachea

3

1.2 Pathology

T. Stadnik, D. De Becker, M. Stienon, and M. Osteaux

The main interest of CT in neoplastic pathology of the neck lies in the precise evaluation of local tumour extension, which is an important factor in therapeutic management. At a later stage, CT allows precise follow-up of the treatment and early detection of recurrence.

Solid, cystic or fatty components of tumours may be characterized by densitometry. CT is the most sensitive method for detection of tumourous calcifications. CT is also helpful in discovering foreign bodies, which are often very difficult to detect with conventional radiography.

The indications for contrast media injection are:
1. Vascular pathology (thrombosis, malformations)
2. The search for adenopathies in lean patients, whose normal anatomical structures are badly outlined because of the lack of fatty interfaces
3. The detection of small laryngeal neoplasms

The contra-indications for iodinated contrast media in thyroid pathology must be kept in mind.

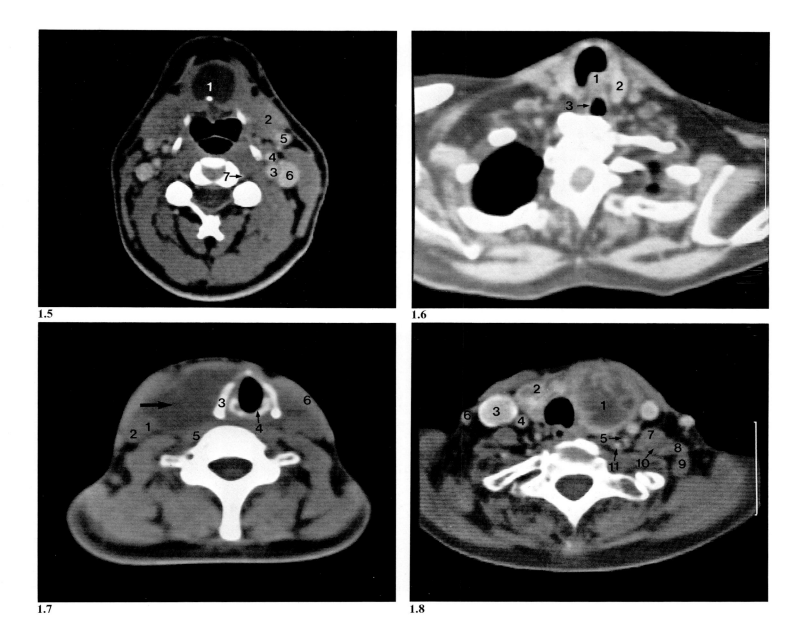

1.5

1.6

1.7

1.8

Fig. 1.5. Thyroglossal cyst. The scan shows medial round cystic formation (*1*) with well-defined outlines in front of the hyoid bone. Unlike in abscesses, there is no contrast enhancement of the cyst wall.

2 Submandibular gland	*5* External jugular vein
3 Internal carotid artery	*6* Internal jugular vein
4 External carotid artery	*7* Vertebral artery

Fig. 1.7. Cervical localization of multiple lymphangioma. The patient presented with a ill-defined semi-fluctuant swelling of the neck and had multiple lymphangiomas of the buccal cavity and the pharynx. The hypodense (30 HU) mass on the right (→) displaces the larynx to the left. Lymphangioma can sometimes form a large multilocular cystic mass.

1 Common carotid artery	*4* Arytenoid cartilage
2 Internal jugular vein	*5* Longus cervicis muscle
3 Thyroid cartilage	*6* Sternocleidomastoid muscle

Fig. 1.6. Tracheal tumour (squamous cell carcinoma). The mass (*1*) protrudes into the tracheal lumen, but spares other structures: the thyroid (*2*) laterally and the oesophagus (*3*) posteriorly. The irregular anterior border of the vertebral body corresponds to arthrosis.

Note that tracheal tumours are difficult to detect using conventional radiographic techniques

Fig. 1.8. Thyroid neoplasia. A 4-mm slice after fast i.v. injection of contrast shows a heterogenous well-encapsulated mass (*1*) of the left lobe with a large central hypodense necrotic area. The heterogeneity in the right lobe indicates infiltration (*2*). The internal jugular vein (*3*), the common carotid artery (*4*) and the trachea are displaced without invasion.

5 Inferior thyroid artery	*9* Scalenus posterior muscle
6 External jugular vein	*10* Brachial plexus
7 Scalenus anterior muscle	*11* Vertebral artery
8 Scalenus medius muscle	

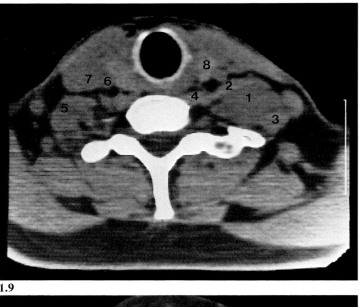

1.9

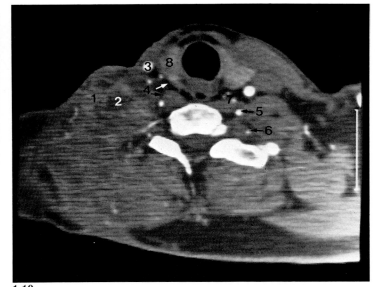

1.10

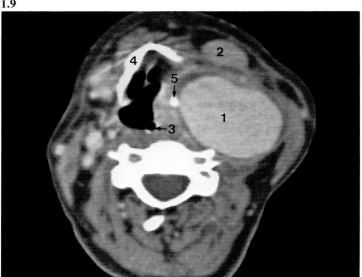

1.11

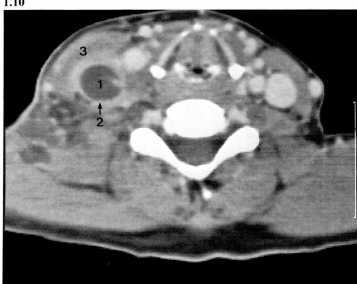

1.12

Fig. 1.9. Neurinoma of the left brachial plexus. The patient complained of pain in the left arm for 8 months. All conventional radiographic examinations were normal. CT shows a mass (*1*) occupying the brachial plexus position, between the scalenus anterior muscle (*2*) and the scalenus medius and posterior muscles (*3*). The low density of the mass is due to its high myelin content.

4 Longus cervicis muscle   *7* Internal jugular vein
5 Right brachial plexus   *8* Thyroid gland
6 Common carotid artery

Fig. 1.11. Carotid artery aneurysm. This section at C4 level was realized with rapid perfusion of contrast medium. The 57-year-old patient had presented with a pulsating mass deforming the neck. There is a significant dilatation of the left common carotid artery (*1*), displacing the laryngeal structures to the right, and a dilatation of the left anterior jugular vein (*2*) corresponding to a collateral pathway due to compression of the internal jugular vein, which is collapsed by the mass and not individualized. Also shown are a gastric sound in the pharynx (*3*), the hyoid bone (*4*) and the upper horn of the thyroid cartilage (*5*)

Fig. 1.10. Recurrence of a surgically treated malignant melanoma. There is infiltration of the whole lateral cervical region. After bolus injection of contrast media (arterial phase) heterogeneity of the mass is evident, with hypervascularized areas (*1*) and with hypovascularized areas (*2*) corresponding to necrosis.

The right common carotid artery (*3*) is displaced but not infiltrated. The fatty tissue (*4* →) between the neoplastic mass, the thyroid gland and the longus cervicis muscle remains unaffected.

5 Vertebral artery   *7* Inferior thyroid artery and
6 Ascending cervical artery   its terminal branches

Fig. 1.12. Internal jugular vein thrombosis. The examination was carried out after perfusion of contrast media; the section is at glottic level. The low density of the lumen of the left internal jugular vein represents a thrombus (*1*), and there is a contrast-enhanced wall around the thrombosed area (*2*). A thrombus usually presents a low-density cast within the lumen of the vessel; however, a fresh thrombus may be isodense with the contrast-enhanced blood and may not be detectable early in its formation. Note the swelling of the sternocleidomastoid muscle (*3*) lateral to the thrombosed vein, due to inflammatory factors

1.3 Larynx and Hypopharynx

S. VUKANOVIC

1.3.1 General Anatomy

The larynx and hypopharynx, constituting the intersection of the respiratory and digestive tracts, belong clinically to the field of otorhinolaryngology.

Anatomically, the larynx is a cartilaginous structure composed of the thyroïd, cricoïd and arytenoïd cartilages and held in place by the ligaments and muscles forming the pharyngolaryngeal inner wall. It is surrounded posteriorly by a semilunar air space, the hypopharynx.

From the clinical point of view, the larynx is divided into three distinct levels: supraglottic, glottic and subglottic. The supraglottic space is delineated inferiorly by the lower margin of the false vocal cords (FVCs), the glottic contains the true vocal cords (TVCs), and the subglottic is defined by the inferior margin of the TVCs and the inferior cricoïd cartilage.

Radiography of the larynx and hypopharynx involves primarily the analysis of soft tissues. Apart from certain air and mucosal interfaces which give high contrast, the essential tissues in this region possess few differences in density.

1.3.2 Role of CT

The majority of pathological processes in the adult larynx and hypopharynx are manifested by alterations in the mucosa. This favours endoscopy as the diagnostic mode, but endoscopy and radiography have complementary roles in the evaluation of pathologies involving the mucosa and the pharyngeal walls at the same time [19, 20, 23, 24, 30, 33, 34].

In our experience, CT has an excellent contribution to make in a routine thorough radiological investigation including xerography, tomography and contrast media examinations. Additional information provided by CT may be vital not only for diagnosis, but also for the design of an optimal therapy [11, 18, 19, 20, 30, 33, 34].

The extra diagnostic security that CT offers can assist in the evaluation of the extent of regional tumour invasion, enabling the choice between surgery and radiotherapy or indeed between radical and conservative surgery [10, 18, 19, 20, 30, 33, 34]. The diagnostic possibilities of CT in trauma-related laryngeal pathologies merit considerable attention [18, 36]. The diagnostic value of CT in trauma cases has already been demonstrated in haematomas, cartilage fractures and iatrogenic lesions following radiotherapy or intubation [18, 35].

The use of CT in the following list of pharyngolaryngeal pathologies has been discussed in the literature, and in our experience the CT scanner has proved its value in all of these indications.

1. Pharyngolaryngeal tumour pathology:
   a) Tumour extension into the pre-epiglottic space or in the paralaryngeal space (tumours at the base of the tongue and at the vallecula of the larynx)
   b) Contralateral submucosal involvement (tumours of FVCs or TVCs)
   c) Tumour extension into the subglottic space, the lumen or the submucosa
   d) Tumour spread into laryngeal cartilage or extralaryngeal tissues
   e) Diagnosis of those laryngeal and pharyngeal lesions which are inaccessible to endoscopy and biopsy (carcinoma evolving from the laryngocele)
   f) Secondary visualization of adenopathies
   g) Tumoral spread of the small tumours of the lateral wall of the piriform sinus: in these cases CT is mandatory for the possibility of partial surgery. However, the majority of the tumours of the hypopharynx are usually assessed by conventional techniques
2. Laryngeal trauma:
   a) Oedema or haematoma obliterating the laryngeal or pharyngeal tissues
   b) Laryngeal cartilage fractures
   c) Iatrogenic traumas (chondronecrosis secondary to radiotherapy or glottal stenosis from intubation)

In these circumstances, the relevant CT explorations offer an appreciation of the traumatic damage, foreseeing obstruction of the respiratory tract and assisting eventual surgical repair [18, 35].

1.3.3 Anatomy and Pathology of Deep Structure of Larynx

1.3.3.1 Preepiglottic Space

The pre-epiglottic space (PES) is situated anteriorly to the normal laryngeal lumen, inaccessible to endoscopy. Invasive conditions often dictate a course of radiotherapy and/or surgery (partial or radical). Anatomically, the PES is constituted essentially of fatty tissue. It is delineated anteriorly by the thyrohyoid membrane and thyroïd cartilage, superiorly by the ligaments of the hyoid and posteriorly by the epiglottic cartilage. These areas constitute the usual sites of tumour invasion (24% of laryngeal tumours, of which half go undiagnosed by clinicians and three-quarters are missed by radiologists using conventional methods [4, 11, 12, 26, 33, 34]).

1.3.3.2 Paraglottic Space

The paraglottic space (PAS) is situated laterally, deep in the larynx, and communicates anteriorly and superiorly with the PES. It lies between the thyroïd cartilage and the quadrangular membrane and is composed primarily of the soft tissues of the fossa along with the TVCs.

Like the PES, this region is a primary target for tumours arising from the FVCs, the ventricles of Morgagni, the TVCs and the pyriform sinus. CT evaluation of tumour invasion is particularly useful in determination of therapy in this area. Of the available radiological techniques, CT scanning is the only way to judge thyroïd cartilage involvement [1, 10, 16, 18, 19, 20, 33].

1.3.3.3 Anterior and Posterior Commissures

The anterior commissure arises from the junction of the vocal ligaments at the inferior boundary of the thyroïd cartilage. At this level the cartilage is separated from the air space by a fine layer of mucosa. On CT, pathological alteration resulting from an infiltrating tumour is seen as thickening of the commissure.

The posterior commissure is formed by the attachment of the vocal cords at the vocal processes of the arytenoïds. Tumour invasion is usually recognized by tumour signs in the soft tissue and displacement towards the medial plane of the arytenoïd cartilages. Tumour spread into this site calls for intensive investigation, checking not only for contralateral invasion, but also for invasion into the subglottic space, as this could radically effect the choice of therapy.

1.3.3.4 Subglottic Space

The subglottic space has the form of an inverted funnel, the perimeter of which consists of mucosa, and the conus elasticus lateraly, and the cricothyroid ligament anteriorly, the lateral crico-aritenoid muscles and the cricoid cartilage. The possibility of submucosal invasion in subglottic cancers merits particular radiological attention because it is often not seen on endoscopy. It is our experience that CT scanning has become the technique of choice for evaluation of malignant subglottic tumour invasion [4, 10, 20, 26, 34].

1.3.4 Conclusion

CT scanning is the most important addition to the radiodiagnostic armoury in the past decade and is revolutionizing modern radiology. Nevertheless, utilization of CT demands evaluation of clinical indications in connection with other complementary radiological techniques [10, 19, 30, 33, 34]. At the time of writing, it has become necessary to define rational courses of behaviour by weighing possible benefits to be gained in patient treatment against the costliness of the procedure.

With these points in mind, it is necessary to determine the practical value of CT among the established methods of investigating pharyngolaryngeal cancers. In two applications CT is essential:
1. The possibility for selective modification of therapeutic treatment (i.e. radiotherapy and partial or radical surgery) in the malignant tumours of the larynx listed above
2. Diagnosis in laryngeal trauma, as already stated in the literature.

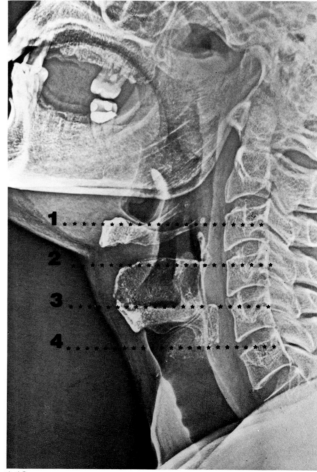

1.13

Fig. 1.13. Xerograph of the neck in a normal subject. Levels 1–4 correspond approximately to the CT sections a–d in Fig. 1.14

8

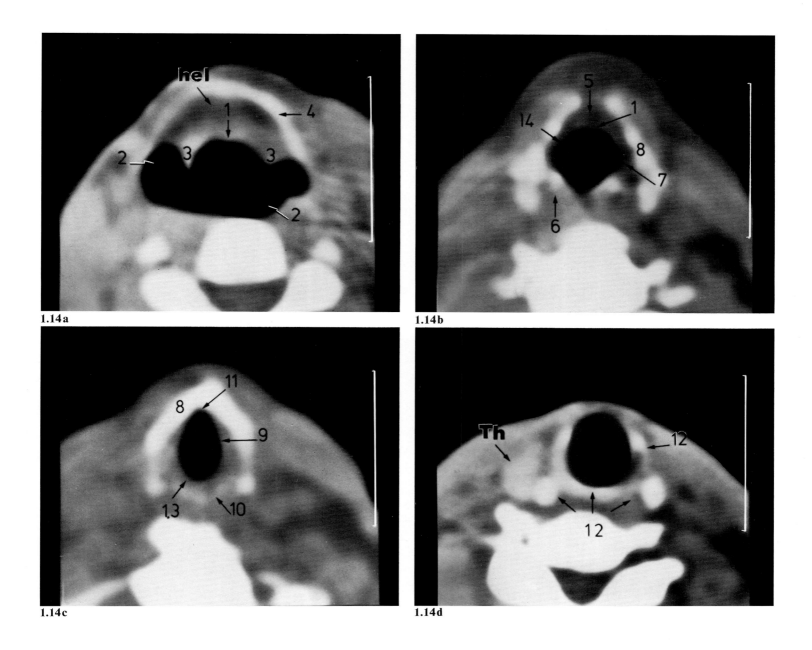

Fig. 1.14a–d. CT scan of the larynx and hypopharynx of a normal subject. **a** Section at the inferior plane of the hyoid bone during Valsalva's manœuvre. **b** Supraglottic section. The two wings of the thyroid (*8*) anteriorly delineate the triangular PES. The posterior FVC (*7*) is also shown. **c** Glottic space section at the plane of the TVCs. At this level two wings of the vocal ligament create an acute angle at their junction (anterior commissure). **d** Subglottic section showing the broad signet portion [19] of the cricoid cartilage (*12*)

1 Epiglottis
2 Hypopharynx
3 Aryepiglottic cords
4 Hyoid cornu
5 PES
6 Cuneiform cartilage
7 FVC
8 Thyroid cartilage

9 TVC
10 Arytenoid cartilage
11 Anterior commissure
12 Cricoid cartilage
13 Posterior commissure
14 PAS
Hel Hyo-epiglottic ligament
Th Thyroid gland

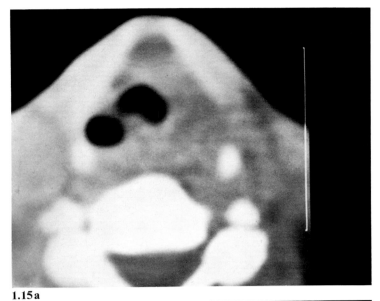

1.15a

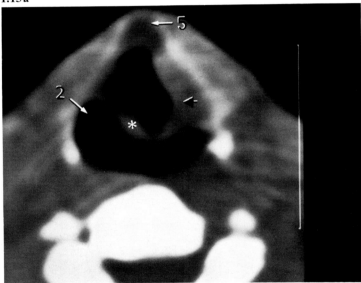

1.15b

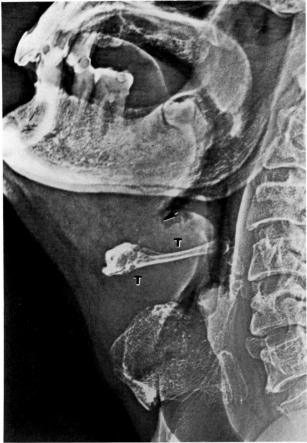

1.16

Fig. 1.15a, b. Demonstration of Valsalva's manœuvre. Both sections are at the same level in the supraglottic space. **a** Without Valsalva's manœuvre. Prolonged inspiration. The laryngeal structures are undiscriminated. **b** With Valsalva's manœuvre. The anatomical structures are clearly and individually visualized.

The FVCs (◄) exhibit thickening of the left cord as a result of tumour infiltration. The hypopharynx (2) is insufflated and its walls are well differentiated. The cuneiform cartilage (∗) and the PES (5) are also shown

Fig. 1.16. Lateral xerograph of an extensive carcinoma (T) situated at the base of the tongue and in the vallecula, with ulceration (*arrow*). Although spread into the PES is rare, due to the protective barrier normally presented by the hyo-epiglottic ligament, it is suspected in this case. The choice of surgical treatment is between hemiglossectomy alone and hemiglossectomy with total laryngectomy. CT is advisable to ascertain the precise extent of tumour invasion, thereby facilitating this decision

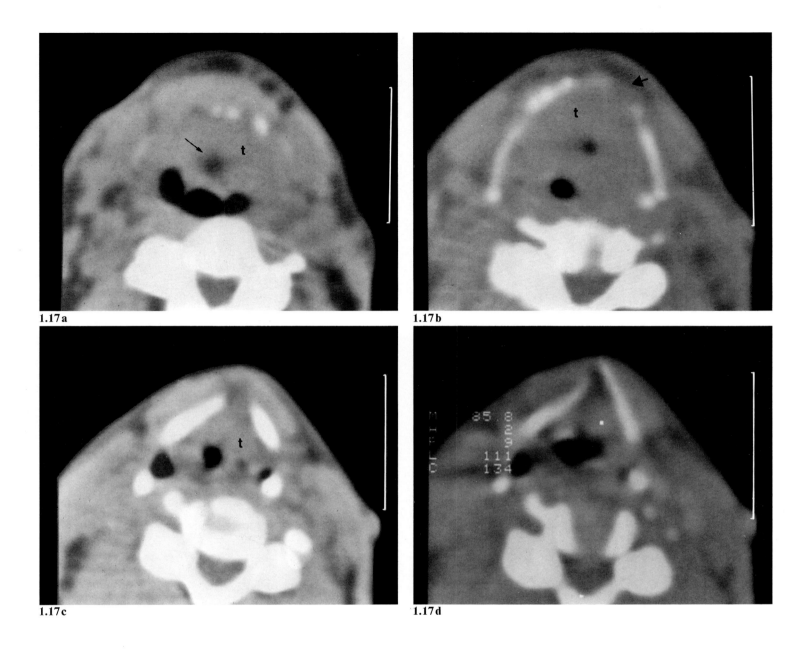

1.17 a

1.17 b

1.17 c

1.17 d

Fig. 1.17. a CT of the oropharynx at the level of the base of the tongue, above the hyoid. The tumour (*t*) is centrally ulcerated (*arrow*). **b** Section at the hyoid plane (8 mm lower than **a**). At this level the tumour (*t*) has extended between the horns of the hyoid bone, invading two valleculae and the epiglottis. The hyoid bone is partially eroded from contact with the tumour (*arrow*). **c** Section at superior supraglottic level. The FVC and the PES have been invaded by the tumour (*t*). **d** Supraglottic section (4 mm lower than **c**) after injection of contrast medium. Tumefaction is restricted to the FVC and PAS.

In this situation a distinction needs to be made between tumour infiltration and peripheral oedema. In this patient, contrast enhancement permitted absolute diagnosis of tumour infiltration (50 HU before and 90 HU after injection of contrast)

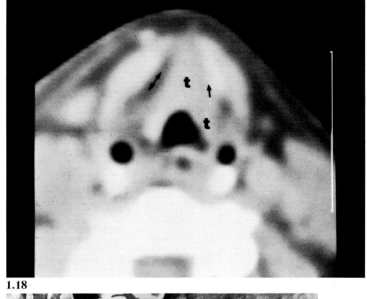

1.18

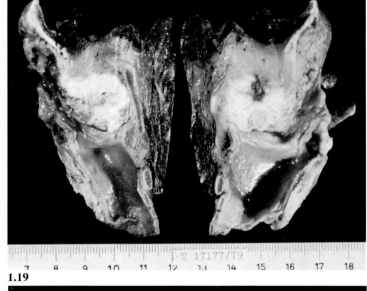

1.19

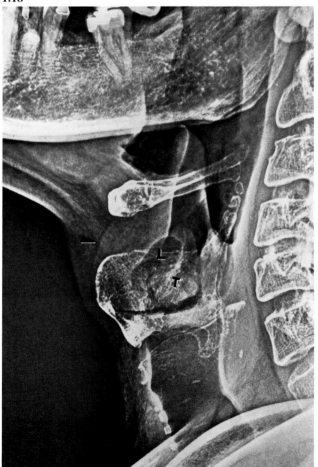

1.20

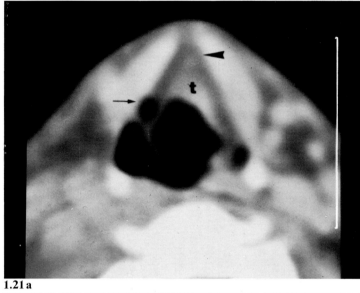

1.21 a

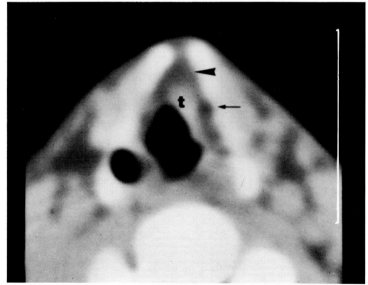

1.21 b

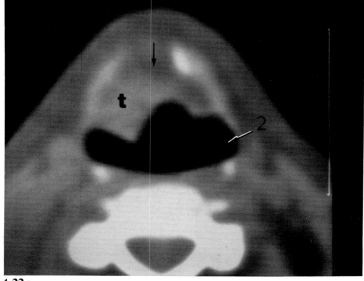

1.22a

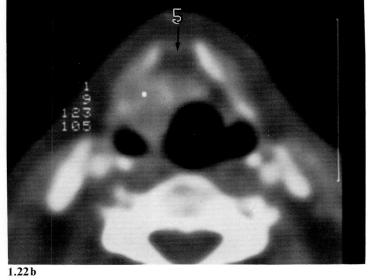

1.22b

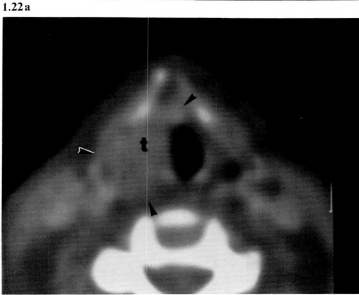

1.22c

1.22d

Fig. 1.22 a–d. Carcinoma of the FVC and of the epiglottis with invasion of the PES. **a** High section of the supra-epiglottic area with Valsalva's manœuvre and without contrast. There is a tumour of the apex of the PES, of the epiglottis and of the PAS on the right (*t*). The anterior portion of the PES is free of tumour (*arrow*). *2*, hypopharynx. **b** Section of the supraglottic area (4 mm lower than **a**) with contrast. The tumour is invading the PES (*5*) and the PAS. The thyroïd cartilage is swollen by the tumour, which seems to extend beyond the cartilage. Posteriorly, the aryepiglottic cord is markedly swollen. After contrast injection the tumour is only slightly enhanced (75 HU before and 93 HU after contrast). **c** Section of the supraglottic area (8 mm below **b**). The tumour (*t*) is eroding the cartilage and invading the hypopharynx (*arrows*). **d** Glottic area section (TVCs) without contrast. Invasion of the posterior third of the right vocal cord (*arrow*) is revealed by CT

◁ **Fig. 1.18.** Carcinoma of the FVCs. The route of invasion was through the PES. The surgical procedure indicated is total laryngectomy. The section is at supraglottic level (plane of the FVCs). There is semilunar infiltration of the right FVC. The tumour (*t*) occupies nearly all the PES and PAS and is confined therein, resting against the cartilage (*single arrow*) but not invading it. On the right is the normal view of the PAS hypodense structure (*doubleheaded arrow*)

Fig. 1.19. Histological confirmation of case shown in Fig. 1.18. Sagittal cross section of the specimen which occupied nearly all the PES, extending to but not invading the cartilage

Fig. 1.20. Carcinoma of the FVC. Lateral xerography demonstrated tumour presence (*t*), but the bilateral laryngoceles (*L*) obscured the PES. Tumour invasion of the PES is a possibility. The *arrow* shows the border of the PES

Fig. 1.21. a As supraglottic section demonstrates that the tumour (*t*) has invaded the FVC laterally and anteriorly, but the PES is not involved (*large arrow*). Laryngocele is seen at opposing angles (*small arrows*). **b** A section 8 mm below **a** demonstrates tumefaction of the left FVC. The PES (*large arrow*) is not involved. The *small arrow* indicates the laryngocele. This patient underwent conservative surgery following CT examination

13

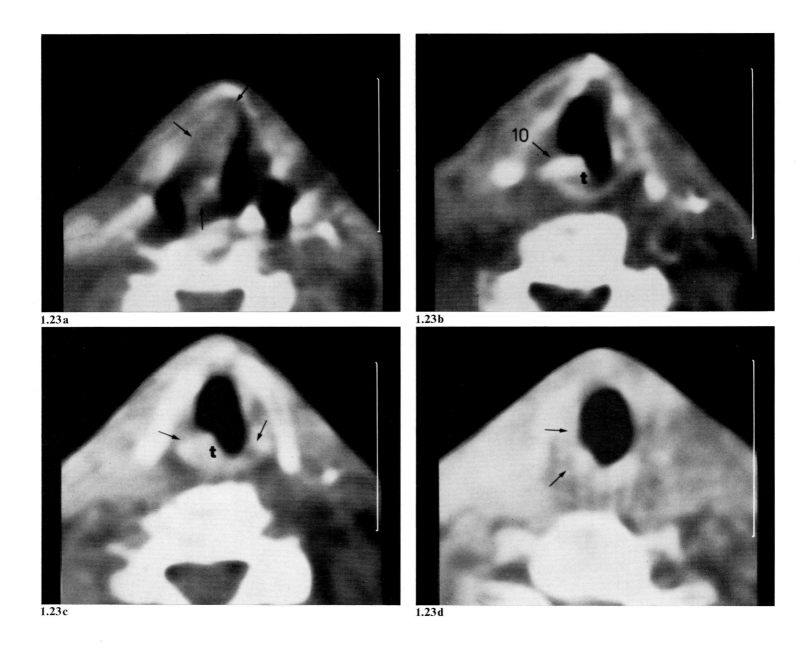

1.23 a

1.23 b

1.23 c

1.23 d

Fig. 1.23 a–d. Carcinoma of the three levels of the glottis. The tumour is invading the posterior commissure on the right and the infraglottic space on the right and posteriorly. CT revealed the infraglottic lesion not seen endoscopically. **a** Section of the supraglottic area without contrast: view of the FVCs. There is marked thickening of the whole of the right FVC with anterior contralateral extension (*arrows*). The tumour does not affect the thyroïd cartilage. **b** Section at the level of the glottis and the anterior commissure without contrast. Thicken- ing of the posterior third of the vocal cord and the posterior com- missure (*t*) is evident. The arytenoïd cartilage (*10*) is displaced anteri- orly and medially by the tumour. **c** Section at the level of the glottis and the lower part of the vocal cords. The tumour (*t*) extends to the posterior circumference, involving the right cord (*arrows*). **d** Sec- tion at infraglottic level. The thickening remains on the right (*arrows*), but the left wall of the lower glottis is again normal. Note the radial artefacts (see text)

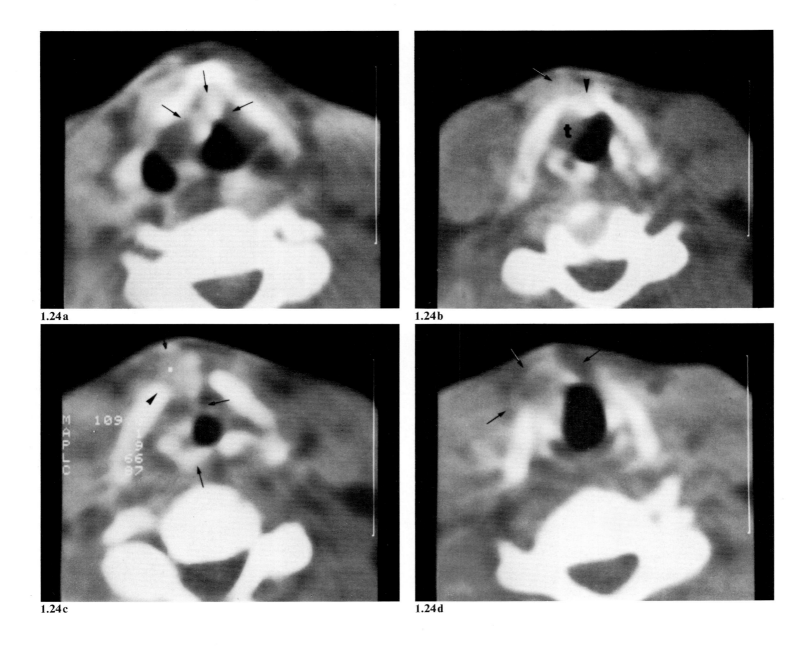

Fig. 1.24 a–d. Carcinoma involving the three laryngeal spaces. This situation particularly indicates CT, as the clinician is unable to view the PES or possible submucosal infiltration of the subglottic space. **a** Supraglottic section revealing invasion (*arrows*) in the thyro-epi-glottic ligament region. **b** Section at the plane of the TVCs. The tumour (*t*) has invaded the TVCs to the right of the anterior com-missure (*arrow*) and the thyroid cartilage (*large arrow*). **c** Section at the inferior margin of the TVCs. There is evident anterior inferior circumferential invasion of the anterior commissure and thyroid carti-lage (*large arrow*). **d** The tumour has invaded the soft tissues (*arrows*) between the cricoid and thyroïd cartilages

15

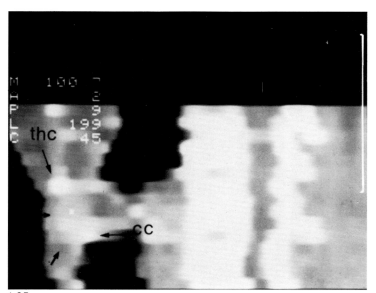

1.25

Fig. 1.25. Medial sagittal reconstruction shows evident anterior tumour invasion (*arrows*) at the base of the epiglottis and extending to the anterior commissure, the TVCs and between the cricoid (*cc*) and thyroid (*thc*) cartilages

Fig. 1.26 a–d. A case of glottic stenosis following prolonged intubation (myasthenia laryngis). **a** Glottic section. The TVCs are fixed with constriction of the cartilages, which are slightly calcified. The *arrowhead* indicates chondronecrosis. *8*, thyroid cortilage. **b–d** Subglottic section showing severe stenois of the subglottic space. The arytenoïd cartilages (*10*) are drawn towards the medial plane (*arrows*). The cricoïd cartilage (*12*) is ruptured and invaded by fibrosis with probable chondronecrosis

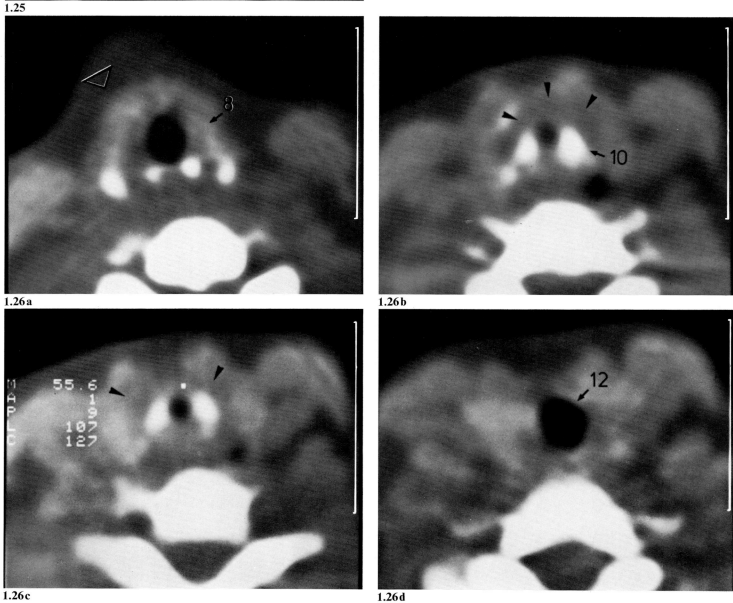

1.26a

1.26b

1.26c

1.26d

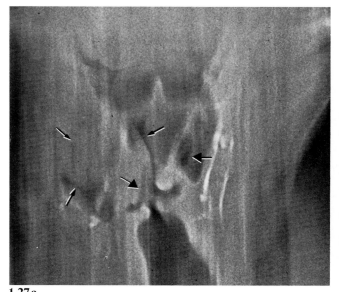

1.27 a

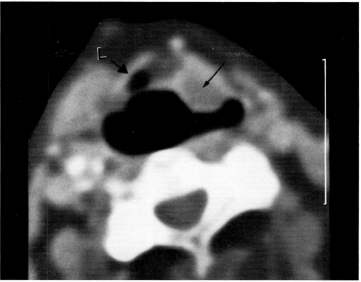

1.27 b

Fig. 1.27 a, b. Tumefaction of the left FVC. Biopsy was negative. Xerography demonstrates an enormous left FVC tumefaction (*small arrows*) and bilateral laryngoceles (*large arrows*). The left laryngocele is compromised by the tumour. Is it a solid tumour in the laryngocele or is there other pathology? CT at the supraglottic space shows an oval encapsulated tumour (*arrow*). The capsule has significant uptake of the contrast medium (60–70 HU); however, the interior remains essentially unchanged (30 HU). Conclusion: abscess corresponding to the cystic formation

References

1. Archer CR, Yeager VL (1979) Evaluation of laryngeal cartilage by CT. J Comput Assist Tomogr 3:604–611
2. Archer CR, Yeager VL, Friedmann W, Katsanonis G (1978) Computed tomography of the larynx. J Comput Assist Tomogr 2:404–411
3. Archer CR, Sagel SS, Yeager VL, Martin S, Friedmann WH (1980) Staging of carcinoma of the larynx: comparative accuracy of CT and laryngography. AJR 136:571–575
4. Baclaisse F (1949) Carcinoma of the larynx. Br J Radiol (suppl 3)
5. Bao-Shan Jing (1978) Malignant tumors of the larynx. Radiol Clin North Am 16:247–260
6. Carter BL, Ignatow SB (1977) Neck and mediastinal angiography by CT scan. Radiology 122:515–516
7. Di Guglielmo L, Campani R, Grabagna P, Mira (1977) La xérographia in otorino laringolatia. Excerpta Medica, Amsterdam
8. Doust BD, Ting VM (1974) Xerography of the larynx. Radiology 110:727–730
9. Fletcher GH, Jing BS (1968) The head and neck, an atlas of tumor radiology. Chicago Year Book Medical Publishers
10. Fraser FR, Abramovich SJ, Houang MB (1980) The clinical application of computed tomography in the assessment of laryngopharyngeal carcinoma (preliminary report). J Laryngol Otol 94:441–448
11. Gaillard J, Mereau P (1953) La loge hyo-thyro-epiglottique, son intérêt dans l'évolution et le traitement des cancers pharyngolaryngés. J Fr Otorhinolaryngol 2:139
12. Gamsu, Webb WR, Shallit JB, Moss AA (1981) CT in carcinoma of the larynx and pyriform sinus: value of phonation scans. AJR 136:577–584
13. Gould LV, Cummings CW, Rabuzzi DD, Reed GF, Chung CT (1977) Use of CAT of the head and neck region. Laryngoscope 87:1270–1276
14. Howell TR, Gildensleene A, King GR (1968) The role of roentgenographic studies in the evaluation and staging of malignancies of the larynx and pharynx. Am J Roentgenol 108:138–144
15. Kirchner JA, Som ML (1971) Clinical significance of fixed vocal cord. Laryngoscope 81:1029–1044
16. Mancuso AA, Hanafee WN (1979) A comparative evaluation of CT and laryngography. Radiology 133:131–138
17. Mancuso AA, Hanafee WN (1979) Computed tomography of the injured larynx. Radiology 133:139–144
18. Mancuso AA, Hanafee WN (1979) Computed tomography and laryngography. Radiology 133:131–138
19. Mancuso AA, Calcaterra TC, Hanafee WN (1978) Computed tomography of the larynx. Radiol Clin North Am 16:195–208
20. Mancuso AA, Hanafee WN, Juillard JF et al. (1977) The role of computed tomography in the management of cancer of the larynx. Radiology 124:243–244
21. Mancuso AA, Tamakawa Y, Hanafee WN (1980) CT of fixed cord. AJR 135:529–534
22. Micheau C, Luboinski B, Sancho H, Cachin Y (1976) Modes of invasion of cancer of the larynx. A statistical, histological and radioclinical analysis of 120 cases. Cancer 38(7):346–360
23. Momose KJ, MacMillan SA (1978) Roentgenologic investigations of the larynx and trachea. Radiol Clin North Am 16:321–341
24. Montgomery WW Surgery of the upper respiratory system. Lea & Febiger, Philadelphia
25. Ogura JH, Heereman H (1973) Conservation surgery of the larynx and hypopharynx. Can J Otolaryngol 2:11–16
26. Olofsson J, Renouf JHP, Van Nostrand AW (1973) Laryngeal carcinoma correlation of roentgenography and histopathology.

A study based on whole organ, serially sectioned laryngeal carcinoma specimens. Am J Roentgenol 117:526–539

27. Patel S, Brennan J (1981) Diagnosis of internal jugular vein thrombosis by CT. J Comput Assist Tomogr 5:197–200
28. Peterson RR (1980) A cross-sectional approach to anatomy. Chicago Year Book Medical Publishers
29. Pressman JJ (1960) Anatomical studies related to the dissemination of cancer of the larynx. Trans Am Acad Ophthalm-Otolaryngol 64:628–638
30. Sagel SS, AufderHeide FJ, Aronberg JD, Stanley JR, Archer RC High resolution computed tomography in the staging of carcinoma of the larynx. The Laryngoscope 91:292–300
31. Som PM, Shugar JMA, Drazin D, Biller HF (1981) Some CT findings in occult thyroid disease. J Comput Assist Tomogr 5:516–518
32. Kaneko T, Matsumoto M, Fukui K, Hori T, Katayama K (1979) Clinical evaluation of thyroid CT values in various thyroid conditions. J Comput Assist Tomogr 3:1–4
33. Vukanovic S, Ducommun JC, Panosetti E (1981) La tomodensitométrie dans la pathologie ORL. Méd et Hyg 39:3694–3705
34. Vukanovic S, Lehmann W, Ducommun JC, Hauser H, Wettstein P (1980) The value of Roentgenographic study (CT and xerography) in the staging of carcinoma of the larynx and hypopharynx. Neue Aspekte radiologischer Diagnostik und Therapie. Jahrbuch SGRNM 1980, Huber, p 50–55
35. Vukanovic S, Sidani AH, Ducommun JC, Suter P, Wettstein P (1982) Tracheal and subglottic lesions following long-standing intubation. A radiological and clinical study. Diagn Imaging 51:224–233
36. Ward PM, Hanafee WN, Mancuso A, Shallit J, Berci G (1979) Evaluation of CT, cinelaryngoscopy and laryngography in determination of the extent of laryngeal disease. Ann Otol Rhinol Laryngol 88:454–462

CHAPTER 2

Lungs

W. Döhring

2.1 Indications

The standard methods for in vivo assessment of morphological pulmonary abnormalities are conventional non-invasive radiographic techniques. In selected cases CT can provide useful additional information and replace invasive examination procedures. Despite limited spatial resolution (1–2 mm) and relatively long scan times (1–5 s), improved detail detectability is obtained by the summation-free representation of transverse sections and increased contrast resolution (0.2–0.5%). Whereas conventional radiography enables the detection of small dense lesions down to 4–5 mm, preferably in central areas of the lung, CT permits the recognition of less dense and still smaller lesions down to 2–3 mm in any part of the lung. The bronchial tree can be evaluated down to the segmental bronchi, abnormal lung vessel distributions can be recognized and a tissue characterization of pulmonary masses (e.g. fat-free soft tissue, fat, fluid, blood, gas inclusions, calcifications), as well as quantitative regional studies of the pulmonary ventilation, can be performed. The following special applications for pulmonary CT scans have proved their usefulness:

a) Investigation of lung regions which cannot be evaluated sufficiently by conventional radiographic techniques (subpleural, paramediastinal, retrosternal, paravertebral and retrocardial lung regions, lung apices and costophrenic angles)
b) Differentiation between parenchymal and pleural processes (e.g. abscess vs empyema, atelectasis vs effusion, emphysematous bulla vs pneumothorax)
c) Staging and treatment planning of bronchial carcinoma (complementary to bronchoscopy and mediastinoscopy)
d) Evaluation of pulmonary nodules (detection of small peripheral nodules, identification of intranodular calcifications)
e) Analysis of cavitary lesions
f) Complementing of conventional radiographic techniques in detecting the spatial distribution of parenchymal lesions and in evaluating hilar, bronchial and vascular abnormalities (e.g. small hilar lymph nodes, bronchiectases, vascular displasiae and arteriovenous aneurysms)
g) Early recognition of diffuse lung diseases and disorders (e.g. incipient pulmonary fibroses, sarcoidosis, lymphangitic metastatic diseases, chronic obstructive lung diseases and fluid overload)
h) Guidance for transthoracic needle biopsies (complementary to fluoroscopy in the case of small processes and difficult locations)
i) Quantitative analysis of regional pulmonary ventilation.

2.2 Technique

Scanning technique (choice of area of interest, slice thickness, slice intervals, scan time, displayed scan field diameter, body position and respiratory phase, application of contrast media) depends on the particular clinical problem to be solved. For detailed examinations of small pulmonary structures, the smallest available slice thicknesses (2–4 mm) should be used in order to reduce partial volume effects. Lung scans must be performed in reproducible constant respiratory phases, e.g. after normal deep inspirations. The respiratory phases can be monitored by means of a spirometer and if necessary can be established exactly with the aid of a shutter valve.

For studies of the regional pulmonary ventilation it is expedient to obtain CT scans at different overall lung volumes, e.g. at total lung capacity, functional residual capacity and residual volume. However, in such examinations it must be taken into consideration that changes of respiratory phase will cause a shift of different lung regions with reference to the fixed scanning plane.

High-speed CT systems enable time-dependent perfusion studies after i.v. bolus injection of uro-angiographic contrast medium (e.g. after bolus injections of 0.5–1 ml of a 30% iodine-containing contrast agent/kg body weight within 3–8 s into a cubital vein).

2.3 Display of Scans

The CT values (expressed in Hounsfield units) of pathological pulmonary structures can vary widely, extending from about −1,000 (e.g. emphysematous bulla) to approximately +1,000 (e.g. calcified metastasis of an osteogenic sarcoma). Therefore in evaluations of pulmonary CT scans, the so-called window (the CT value interval which is displayed in grey steps or colours) must be varied accordingly in both level and width. Generally, window widths of 500 to 1,000 HU and window levels of -600 to -900 HU are used to examine ventilated lung parenchyma; non-ventilated lung tissue requires higher window levels of about 0 to $+50$ HU. Optimal visualization of bronchi is obtained with window widths of about 1,500 to 2,000 HU and window levels in the range of -100 to -600 HU.

Due to the limited spatial resolution of CT systems, the represented diameter of structures within the air-containing lung parenchyma depends on the chosen window level and to a smaller extent on the window width. Thus, for example, with window settings suitable for the assessment of ventilated lung tissue the diameters of blood vessels, cavity walls and pulmonary nodules are represented too large and the diameters of tracheal and bronchial lumina too small.

2.4 Scanners and Recording Conditions

The CT images presented in this chapter were produced using the Somatom and Somatom SF rotating fan beam CT systems (Siemens AG). The following scanning parameters were selected: tube voltage 125 kV, mAs product 230, scan time 5 s, matrix size 256×256, displayed scan field diameter 27–36 cm. The individually chosen slice thicknesses and window settings are specified in the figure legends. Usually the tomograms were taken during breathholding after normal deep inspiration.

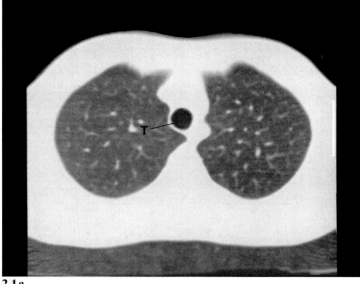

2.1 a

2.1 b

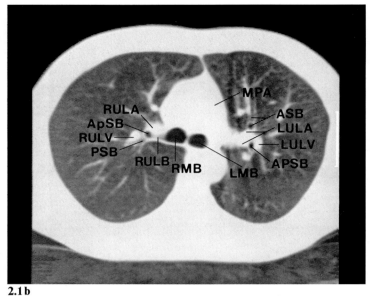

2.1 c

2.1 d

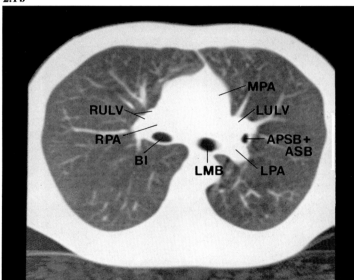

Fig. 2.1 a–h. Normal cross-sectional anatomy of the lungs, demonstrated by means of eight key sections. Slice thickness (S) 8 mm; window width (WW) 1,500 HU; window level (WL) −800 HU. **a** Section at the level of the trachea. **b** Section through the main bronchi. The upper portion of the left hilum can assume highly variable configurations concerning bronchial branching and vascular coursing. In the present case the left anterior segmental bronchus shows an atypical apico-anterior extension. **c** Section through the right upper lobe bronchus. **d** Section through the bronchus intermedius. Under normal conditions the posterior walls of the right main bronchus and the right upper lobe bronchus, as well as the posterior and posteromedial walls of the bronchus intermedius, are in direct contact with lung parenchyma representing the azygo-oesophageal recess. **e** Section through the left upper lobe bronchus. The posterior wall of the left upper lobe bronchus is often slightly indented by the left interlobar artery (see Fig. 2.47); this indentation should not be mistaken for a pathological bronchial narrowing. **f** Section through the middle lobe bronchus. **g** Section through the origins of the superior segmental bronchi. **h** Section through basal segmental branches of the lower lobe bronchi.

The tracheobronchial tree can be readily identified down to its segmental branches; occasionally even initial parts of subsegmental branches are visible (**b, c, f**). In general the hilar arteries and veins show constant relations to the central bronchial tree; their clear identification therefore requires i.v. bolus injections of contrast medium only in particular cases.

The oblique fissures can often be visualized (**c, h;** → →), especially when they are scanned at small slice thicknesses (e.g. Fig. 2.14). The horizontal fissure cannot be visualized.

At inspiratory overall lung volumes the normal respiratory parenchyma is almost homogeneously ventilated; during expiration the increasing lung density usually shows a gravity-dependent gradient (see Fig. 2.10a, b).

T	Trachea
RMB	Right main bronchus
LMB	Left main bronchus
RULB	Right upper lobe bronchus
LULB	Left upper lobe bronchus

22

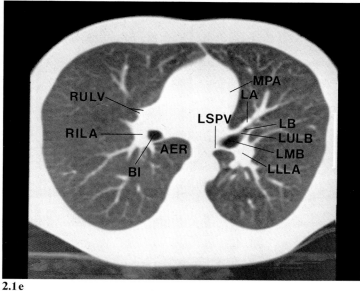

2.1 e

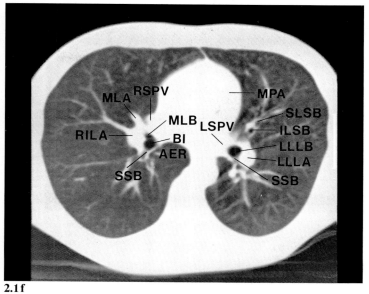

2.1 f

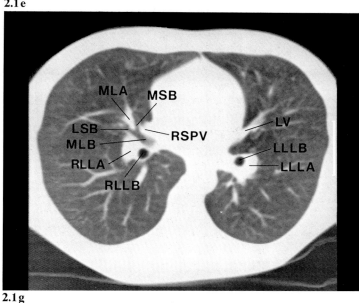

2.1 g

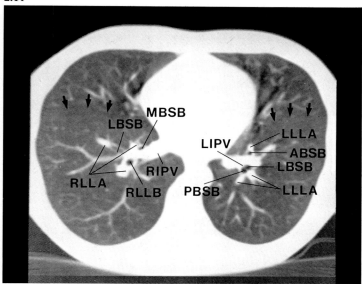

2.1 h

BI	Bronchus intermedius	*RPA*	Right pulmonary artery
MLB	Middle lobe bronchus	*LPA*	Left pulmonary artery
LB	Lingular bronchus	*TA*	Truncus anterior
RLLB	Right lower lobe bronchus	*RILA*	Right interlobar artery
LLLB	Left lower lobe bronchus	*RULA*	Right upper lobe arteries
ApSB	Apical segmental bronchus	*LULA*	Left upper lobe arteries
PSB	Posterior segmental bronchus	*MLA*	Middle lobe artery
APSB	Apical posterior segmental bronchus	*LA*	Lingular artery
ASB	Anterior segmental bronchus	*RLLA*	Right lower lobe arteries
LSB	Lateral segmental bronchus	*LLLA*	Left lower lobe arteries
MSB	Medial segmental bronchus	*RSPV*	Right superior pulmonary vein
SLSB	Superior lingular segmental bronchus	*RULV*	Right upper lobe veins
ILSB	Inferior lingular segmental bronchus	*LSPV*	Left superior pulmonary vein
SSB	Superior segmental bronchus	*LULV*	Left upper lobe veins
MBSB	Medial basal segmental bronchus	*LV*	Lingular vein
ABSB	Anterior basal segmental bronchus	*RIPV*	Right inferior pulmonary vein
LBSB	Lateral basal segmental bronchus	*LIPV*	Left inferior pulmonary vein
PBSB	Posterior basal segmental bronchus	*AOR*	Azygo-oesophageal recess
MPA	Main pulmonary artery		

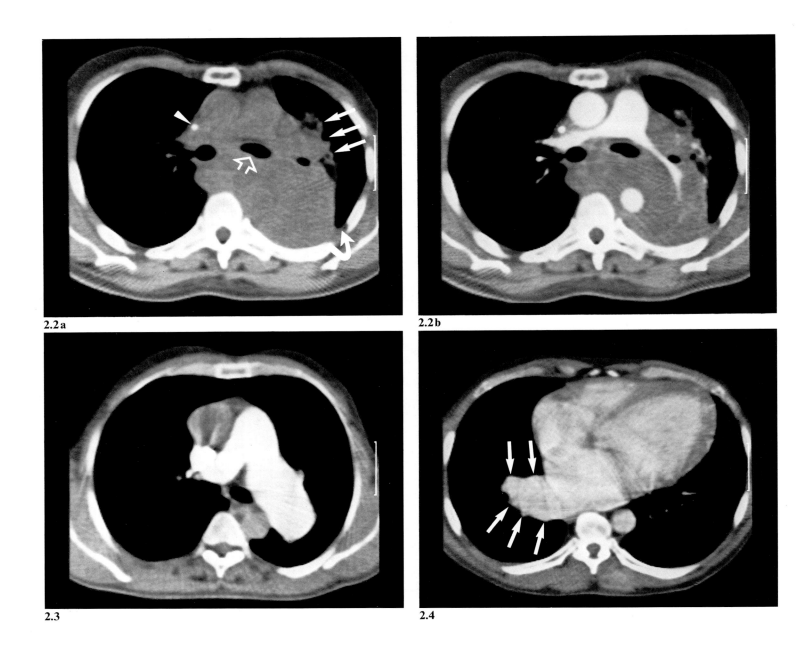

2.2 a

2.2 b

2.3

2.4

Fig. 2.2a, b. Ventral displacement and narrowing of both pulmonary arteries caused by large lymph node metastases from a testicular semi-noma. S 8 mm; WW 512 HU; WL +40 HU. **a** Plain scan; **b** contrast-enhanced scan.

Note furthermore: forward displacement of the ascending aorta and the bronchial tree, tumorous walling in the descending aorta, partial occlusion of the left main bronchus (⇨); compressed lung tissue (→ →); a small left-sided pleural effusion (ↄ); and the catheter in the displaced superior vena cava (►)

Fig. 2.3. Aneurysmal dilatation of the left pulmonary artery caused by pulmonary valvular stenosis. Contrast-enhanced scan. S 8 mm; WW 600 HU; WL +60 HU

Fig. 2.4. Aneurysmal dilatation of the right inferior pulmonary vein (→ →) in chronic mitral valvular disease. Contrast-enhanced scan. S 8 mm; WW 512 HU; WL +85 HU

24

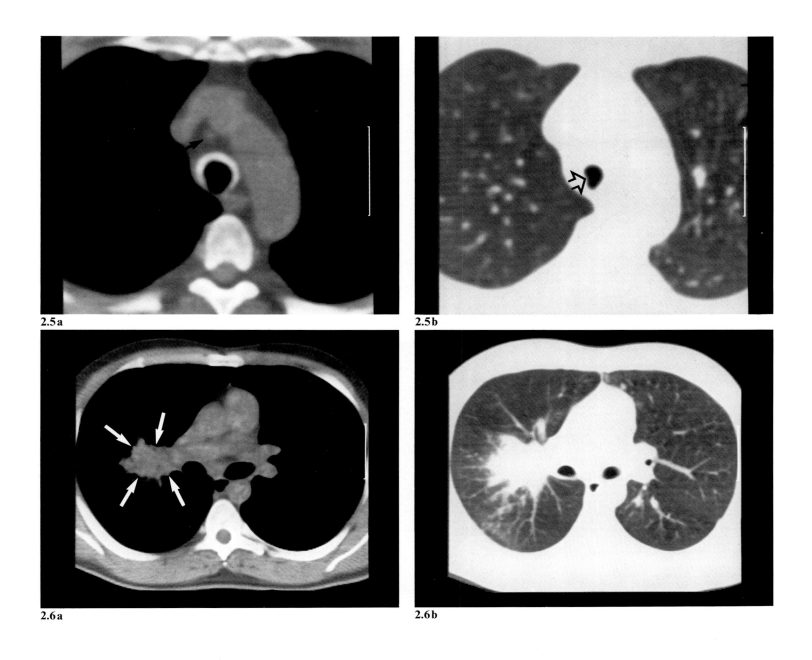

2.5a

2.5b

2.6a

2.6b

Fig. 2.5a, b. Calcification of the tracheal cartilaginous rings. Note the circumscribed mucosal thickening by chronic tracheitis (⇨) and the small pretracheal lymph node (→). **a** S 4 mm; WW 1024 HU; WL +50 HU. **b** Same section; WW 1024 HU; WL −900 HU.

Note the influence of the chosen window width on the diameter of the imaged tracheal lumen

Fig. 2.6a, b. Right hilar lymph node metastases from hypernephroma. **a** S 8 mm; WW 600 HU; WL +50 HU. **b** Same section; WW 1024 HU; WL −850 HU.

There is an irregular mass (→ →) lateral to the right descending pulmonary artery. The accentuation of the bronchovascular structures and the increase in density of the surrounding lung parenchyma indicate lymphatic obstruction with interstitial oedema

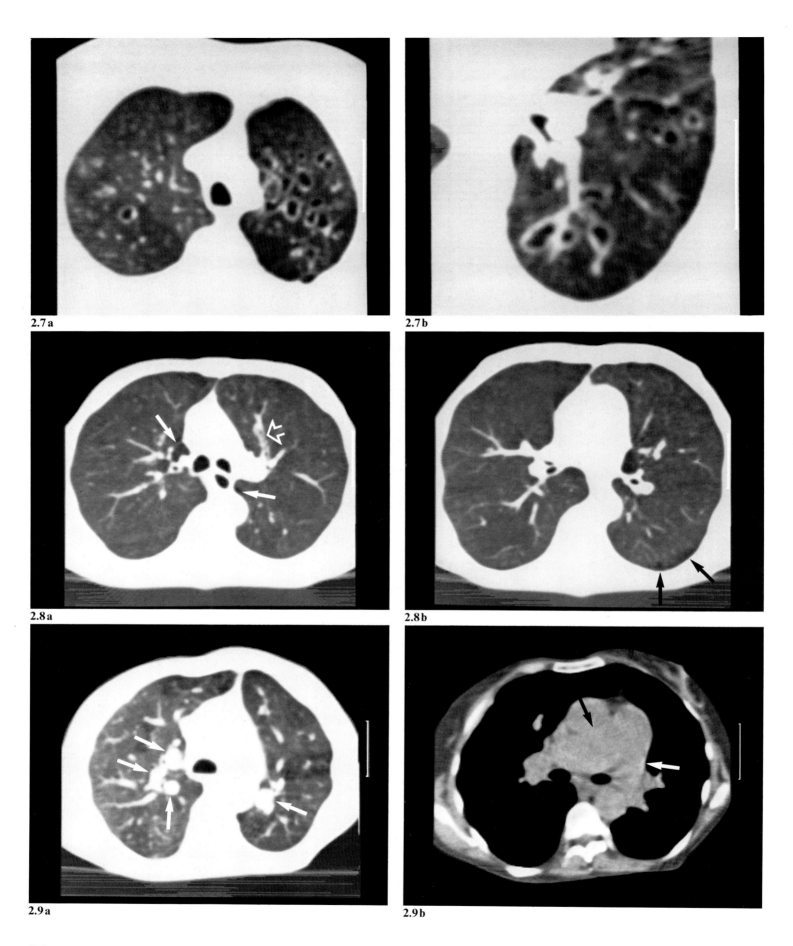

2.7 a

2.7 b

2.8 a

2.8 b

2.9 a

2.9 b

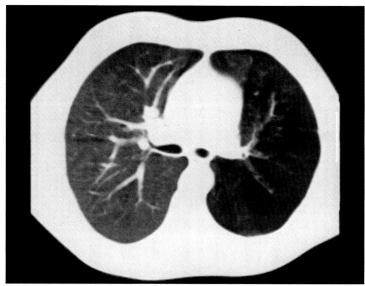

2.10a

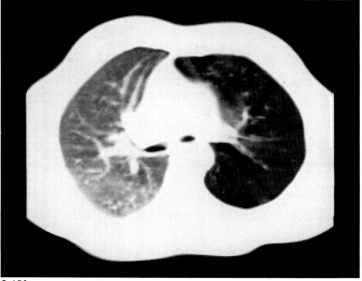

2.10b

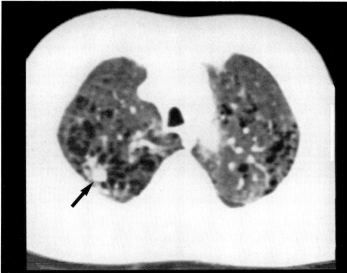

2.11

Fig. 2.10a, b. Unilateral emphysema (Swyer-James' or MacLeod's syndrome). S 8 mm; WW 1024 HU; WL −800 HU. **a** Scan taken after maximal inspiration. **b** Comparable scan taken after maximal expiration.

The two lungs show remarkable differences in density, caused by bronchial obstruction and decreased perfusion of the left lung. There are irregularly shaped segmental bronchi on the left side and severely attenuated central and peripheral left pulmonary vessels. During expiration, air trapping in the left lung causes the mediastinum to move to the right

Fig. 2.11. Emphysematous bullae. S 4 mm; WW 1024 HU; WL −850 HU.

Pericicatrical emphysema with multiple small bullae in both upper lung lobes. The dense peripheral area in the right posterior segment represents a cicatrical carcinoma (→)

◁ **Fig. 2.7a, b.** Bronchiectasis. **a** Ring-shaped densities in the upper lobes of an emphysematous lung, representing ectatic bronchi with thickened walls. S 4 mm; WW 1024 HU; WL −850 HU. **b** Enlarged section of a scan taken from the same lung. There are saccular bronchiectases in the superior segment of the left lower lobe. S 4 mm; WW 800 HU; WL −900 HU

Fig. 2.8a, b. Pulmonary emphysema with generalized overinflation and peripheral vascular deficiency. S 8 mm; WW 1024 HU; WL −800 HU. **a** Section through the main bronchi. **b** Section through the lower lobe bronchi.

Evident are overinflation of both lungs with lowered parenchymal density, small subpleural bullae (→) and diminished peripheral vasculature; sagittally widened chest with reduced diameters of the ventral and dorsal mediastinum; and increased retrosternal lung volume and enlarged azygo-oesophageal recess. The left anterior segmental bronchus is irregularly thickened by chronic bronchitis (⇒)

Fig. 2.9a, b. Chronic obstructive lung disease with severe arterial hypertension (cor pulmonale). **a** Section through the upper lung lobes. S 8 mm; WW 1024 HU; WL −800 HU. **b** Section through the right and left pulmonary arteries. S 8 mm; WW 512 HU; WL +40 HU.

The scan shows inhomogeneously ventilated lungs, with regional overinflations and areas of increased density due to interstitial oedema; dilated central and parahilar pulmonary arteries (→); and irregularly sized and distributed peripheral vessels

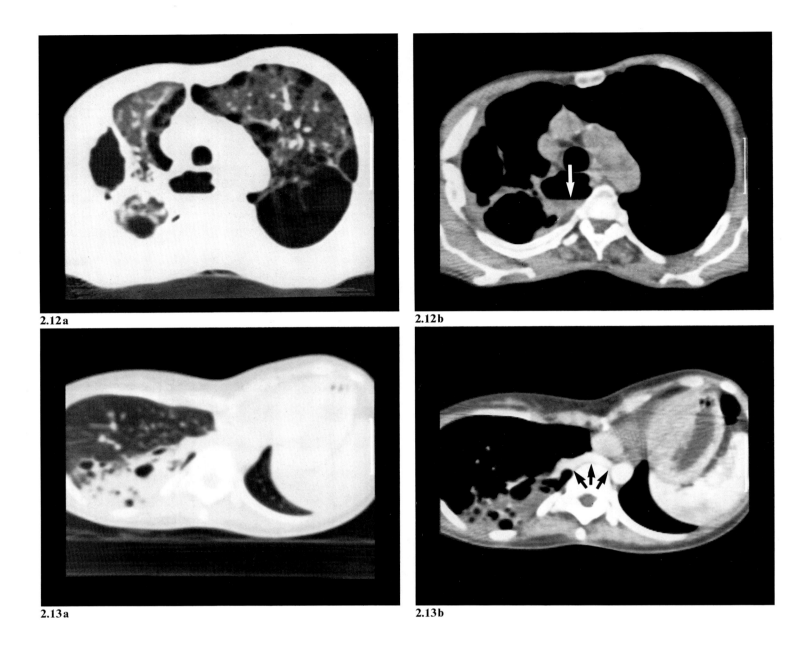

2.12a

2.12b

2.13a

2.13b

Fig. 2.12a, b. Severe bullous emphysema. **a** S 4 mm; WW 1024 HU; WL −900 HU. **b** Same section; WW 600 HU; WL +50 HU.

Multiple bullae of different sizes, predominantly distributed in the peripheral areas of both lungs. An air-fluid level (→) is seen in one of the right pulmonary air sacs. The right-sided posterolateral bullae are surrounded by dense compressed lung tissue and pleural thickenings. Note the asymmetry of the thoracic cross section and the displacement of the mediastinum

Fig. 2.13 a, b. Pulmonary sequestration; funnel chest. **a** Well-defined cystic mass in the posterior portion of the right lower lobe. S 8 mm; WW 2046; WL −600 HU. **b** Enhanced anomalous artery (→) arising from the descending thoracic aorta, running behind the inferior vena cava and supplying the sequestered portion of the lung. S 8 mm; WW 512 HU; WL +50 HU.

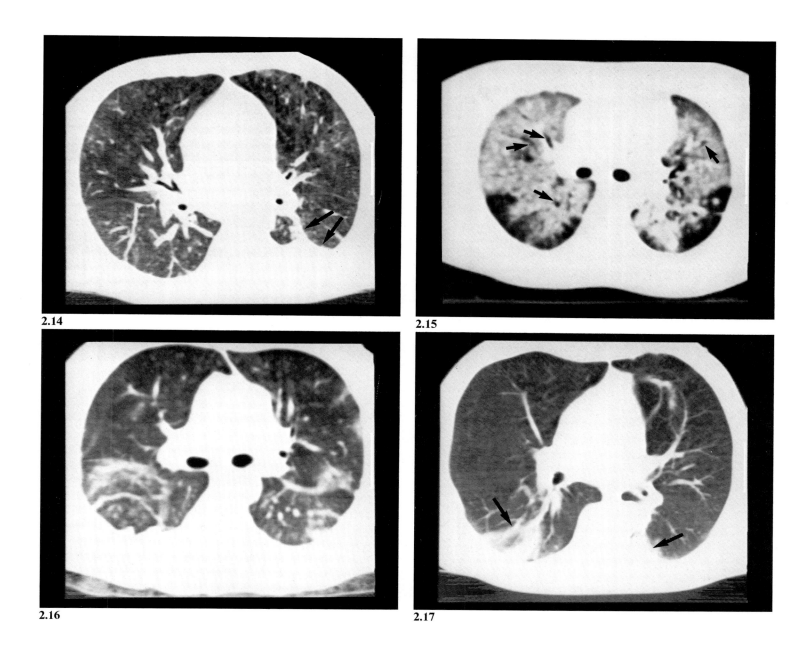

2.14

2.15

2.16

2.17

Fig. 2.15. Predominantly alveolar oedema. S 4 mm; WW 1024 HU; WL −650 HU.

The scan shows confluent, irregular and poorly defined parenchymal consolidations with air bronchograms (→), which extend bilaterally and fairly symmetrically from the hila to the periphery

Fig. 2.14. Interstitial oedema. S 2 mm; WW 1024 HU; WL −800 HU.

There are indistinct areas of increased density and slightly accentuated vascular markings in both lungs, and a small atelectasis and pleural effusion on the left side (→ →)

Fig. 2.16. Pulmonary contusion after blunt chest trauma. S 4 mm; WW 1024 HU; WL −800 HU.

Poorly defined, differently shaped areas of increased density are irregularly distributed over both lungs

Fig. 2.17. Recurrent pulmonary infarctions. S 8 mm; WW 1024 HU; WL −800 HU.

The roughly triangular dense areas in the superior segments of both lower lobes (→) represent pulmonary infarctions; their bases abut upon the pleural surface and their apices are directed towards the hila. The small angular dense area in the lingula is probably also caused by pulmonary embolism

29

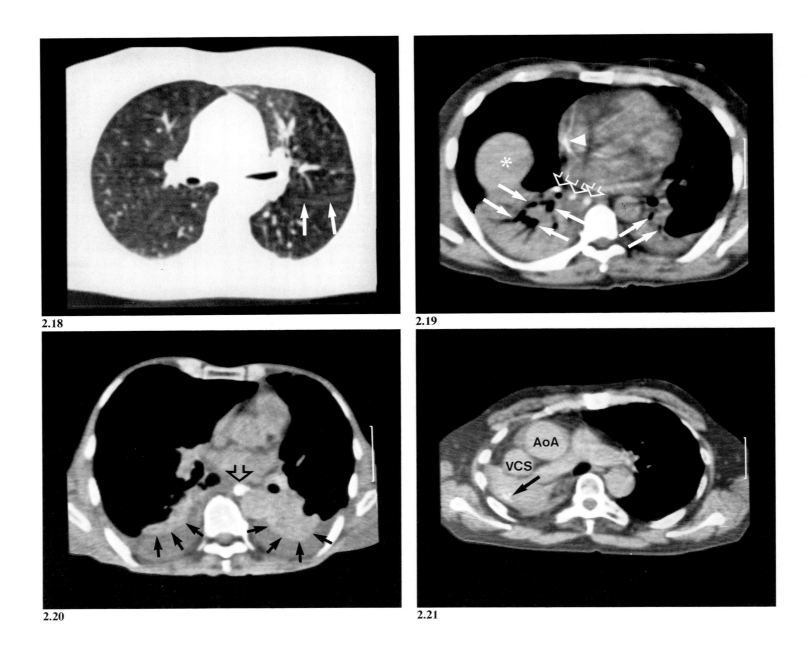

Fig. 2.18. Initial poststenotic atelectasis of the left anterior segment due to bronchial carcinoma. S 4 mm; WW 1024 HU; WL −800 HU.

The less ventilated segment appears increased in density and shrunken towards the mediastinum; the adjacent segments and the left major septum (→ →) are displaced forward

Fig. 2.20. Bilateral paravertebral atelectases and pleural effusions in an artificially ventilated patient. S 4 mm; WW 512 HU; WL + 50 HU.

The borderlines between the dense non-ventilated lung parenchyma and the less dense pleural effusions (→ →) are plainly visible. There is a stomach tube in the oesophagus (⇨)

Fig. 2.19. Complete atelectases of the right lower lobe and the basal segments of the left lower lobe with well-defined longitudinally and transversely sectioned air bronchograms (→). S 8 mm; WW 512 HU; WL +40 HU.

Note the right diaphragmatic dome (∗) and the calcified right hilar lymph nodes (⇨), as well as the catheter in the right atrium (▶)

Fig. 2.21. Total right pulmonary atelectasis in a patient with severe spondylarthritis, chronic bronchitis, treated lung tuberculosis and aortic valvular insufficiency. S 8 mm; WW 512 HU; WL +40 HU.

The scan shows a completely collapsed right lung with reduced right thoracic cross section and displaced mediastinum. There are right pulmonary calcifications (→), the superior vena cava (*VCS*) and the ascending aorta (*AoA*) one dilated

30

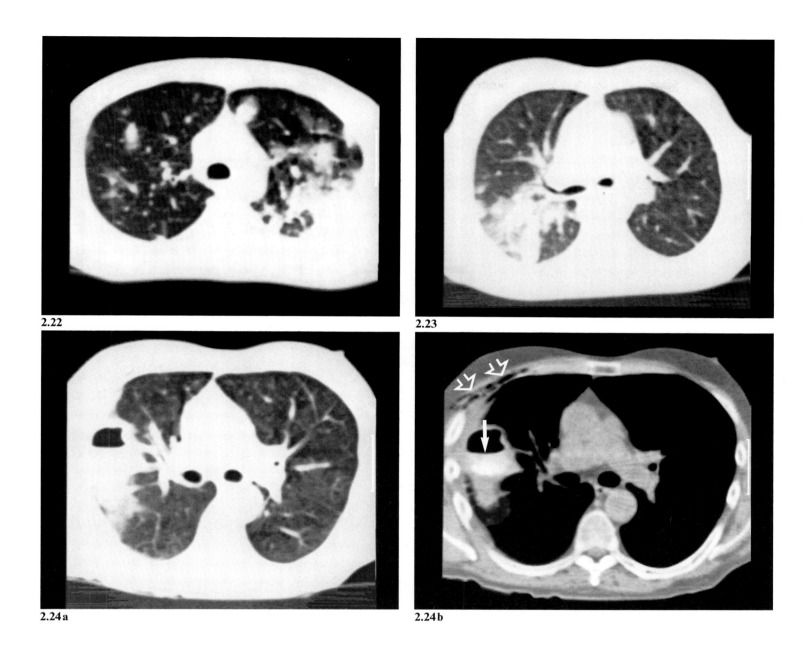

2.22

2.23

2.24 a

2.24 b

Fig. 2.22. Bilateral bronchopneumonia. S 4 mm; WW 1500 HU; WL −500 HU.

Patchy confluent consolidations are scattered over both lungs, and there is a small left-sided pleural effusion

Fig. 2.23. Pneumonia with segmental distribution. S 4 mm; WW 1500 HU; WL −700 HU.

Inhomogeneous inflammatory infiltration affects the posterior segment of the right upper lobe

Fig. 2.24a, b. Pulmonary abscess. **a** S 4 mm; WW 1024 HU; WL −800 HU. **b** Same section; WW 1024 HU; WL 0 HU.

The solitary cavity in the lateral portion of the right upper lobe has a thick dense wall and an air-fluid level (→). The wall is surrounded posteromedially by inflamed lung tissue and bordered laterally by pleural thickenings. The fluid contains the remains of contrast medium injected through the thoracic wall some days before; the injection has caused a circumscribed chest wall emphysema (⇨⇨)

31

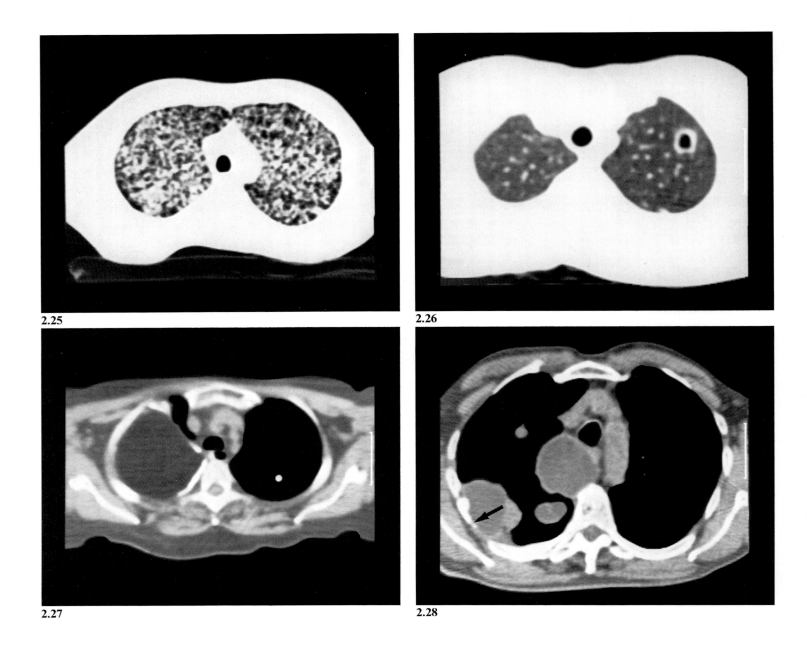

2.25

2.26

2.27

2.28

Fig. 2.25. Miliary pulmonary tuberculosis. S 8 mm; WW 1024 HU; WL −500 HU.

Innumerable tiny, discrete and partly confluent dense areas are spread symmetrically throughout both lungs

Fig. 2.27. Right-sided oleothorax and left-sided tuberculoma. S 8 mm; WW 700 HU; WL +50 HU.

This paraffin plombage is about 40 years old, with calcifications in the ventromedial and dorsomedial walls. The attenuation of the paraffin amounts to −139 ±7.5 HU. The CT values of the calcified tuberculoma exceed +700 HU

Fig. 2.26. Persistent tuberculous cavitation. S 4 mm; WW 800 HU; WL −850 HU.

An air-filled cavity with a dense wall and a fairly smooth surface is shown in the left pulmonary apex

Fig. 2.28. Thoracic echinococcosis. S 4 mm; WW 512 HU; WL +50 HU.

Multiple sharply circumscribed right pulmonary cysts are seen, each with a thin dense wall and a homogeneous fluid content. The CT values of the fluid amount to 10 ±7.3 HU. One cyst has eroded an adjacent rib (→)

32

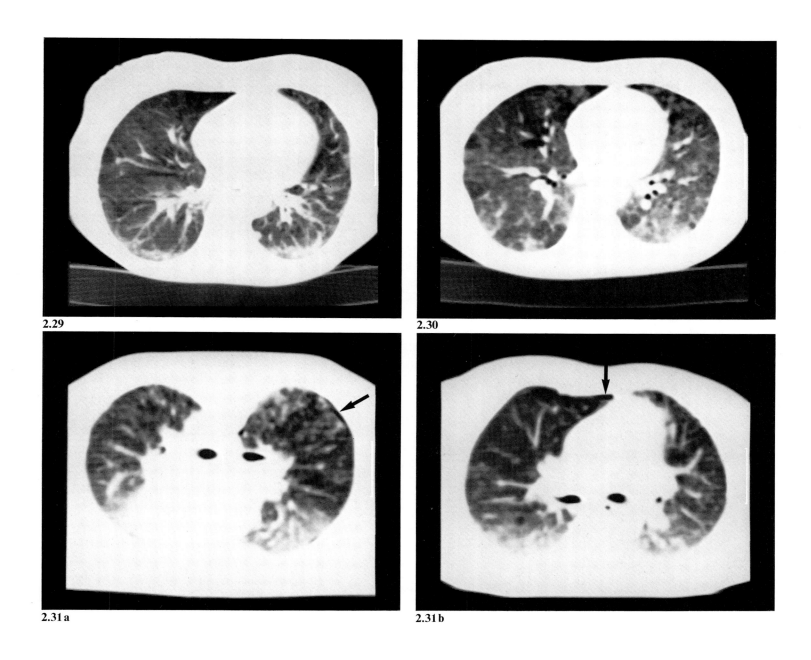

2.29

2.30

2.31 a

2.31 b

Fig. 2.29. Pulmonary fibrosis in scleroderma. S 8 mm; WW 1024 HU; WL −750 HU.

There is a slight increase in pulmonary density. The perivascular densifications are accentuated in the dorsobasal region of each lung

Fig. 2.30. Pulmonary fibrosis with patchy densities, irregular vascularization, reticular structures and honeycomb pattern. S 8 mm; WW 1024 HU; WL −600 HU

Fig. 2.31a, b. Pulmonary fibrosis with predominant reticular pattern scanned in different body positions. S 8 mm; WW 1024 HU; WL −600 HU. **a** Scan in supine position. The small right-sided pneumothorax (→) was caused by a transthoracic needle biopsy. **b** Scan in prone position.

Increases in density of dependent lung regions due to fibrosis and based on gravity effects can be differentiated by comparable scans in different body positions

33

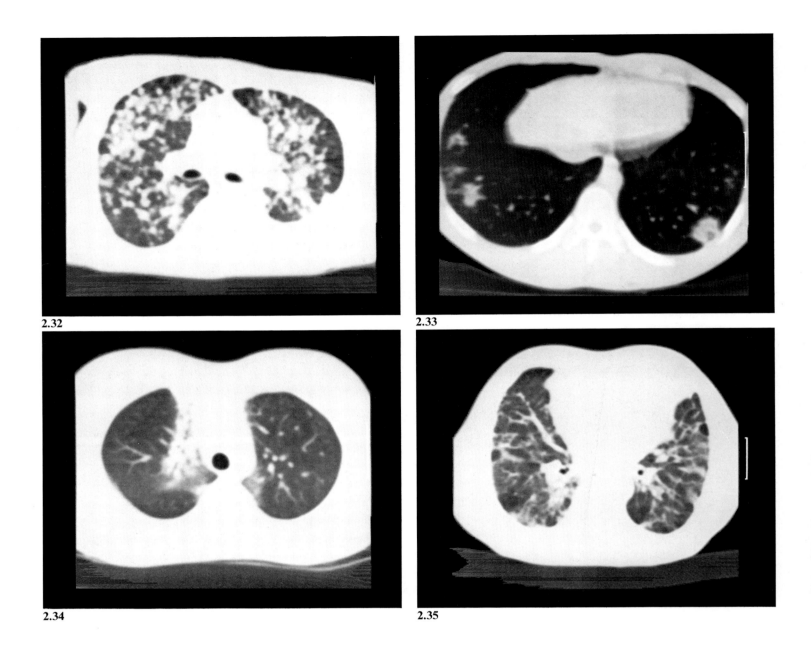

2.32

2.33

2.34

2.35

Fig. 2.32. Pulmonary fibrosis with predominant nodular pattern. S 8 mm; WW 1500 HU; WL −700 HU.

The multiple confluent, small nodules scattered throughout both lungs indicate acinar involvement. Left-sided pleural effusion is evident

Fig. 2.34. Irradiation fibrosis. S 8 mm; WW 1500 HU; WL −700 HU.

There is well-defined right paramediastinal shrinkage. The considerable loss of volume corresponds to an area irradiated because of malignant thymoma

Fig. 2.33. Bleomycin-induced pulmonary fibrosis. S 4 mm; WW 2046 HU; WL −200 HU.

The multiple focal areas of pulmonary fibrosis mimic recurrent metastases in the lower lung regions of a bleomycin-treated patient with testicular carcinoma

Fig. 2.35. Asbestosis. S 8 mm; WW 1500 HU; WL −700 HU.

The late stage of parenchymal manifestation displays coarse reticulation and a honeycomb pattern

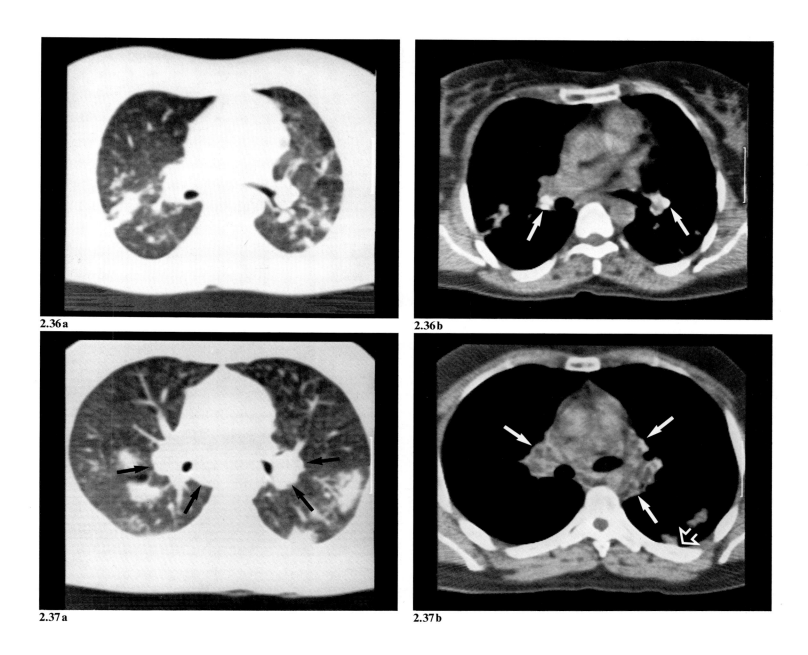

2.36a

2.36b

2.37a

2.37b

Fig. 2.36a, b. Silicosis. **a** S 4 mm; WW 1500 HU; WL −700 HU. **b** Same section; WW 512 HU; WL +50 HU.

Fairly well circumscribed nodules of different sizes and irregular conglomerations of confluent nodules are scattered throughout both lungs, accompanied by fibrosis and regional overinflations. Note the bilateral hilar lymph node calcifications (→)

Fig. 2.37a, b. Sarcoidosis. **a** Involvement of lung parenchyma. S 8 mm; WW 1024 HU; WL −800 HU. **b** Mediastinum and pulmonary hila. S 8 mm; WW 512 HU; WL +40 HU.

There are clustered granulomas in both lungs, with pleural involvement (⇒) on the left side. The mediastinal and bilateral hilar lymph nodes are enlarged (→)

35

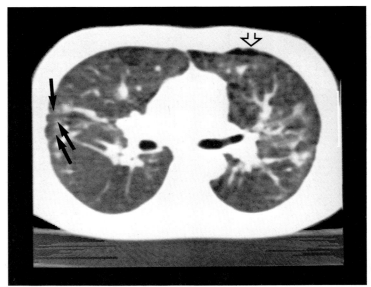

2.38

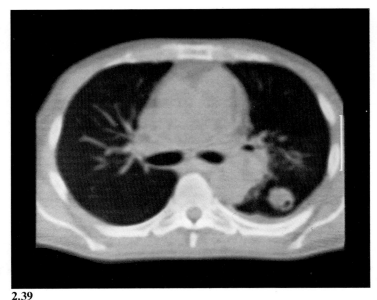

2.39

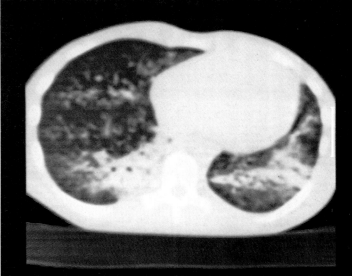

2.40

Fig. 2.38. Sarcoidosis with pulmonary fibrosis. S 4 mm; WW 1024 HU; WL −800 HU.

Irregular vascularization, patchy densities and coarse fibrotic strands extending from both hila to the periphery are seen, along with thickened interlobular septa (→) with tiny pleural spikes, and small subpleural overinflations (⇒)

Fig. 2.39. Wegener's granulomatosis. S 8 mm; WW 1800 HU; WL −100 HU.

The scan shows a rounded cavitated density in the superior segment of the left lower lobe rather poorly defined parenchymal consolidation in the left parahilar region and a small left-sided pleural effusion

Fig. 2.40. Goodpasture's syndrome. S 8 mm; WW 1800 HU; WL −500 HU.

A section through the lower lung regions taken during an acute episode of pulmonary haemorrhage shows mottled opacities and areas of major air-space consolidations in both lungs with cross-sectioned air bronchograms on the right side

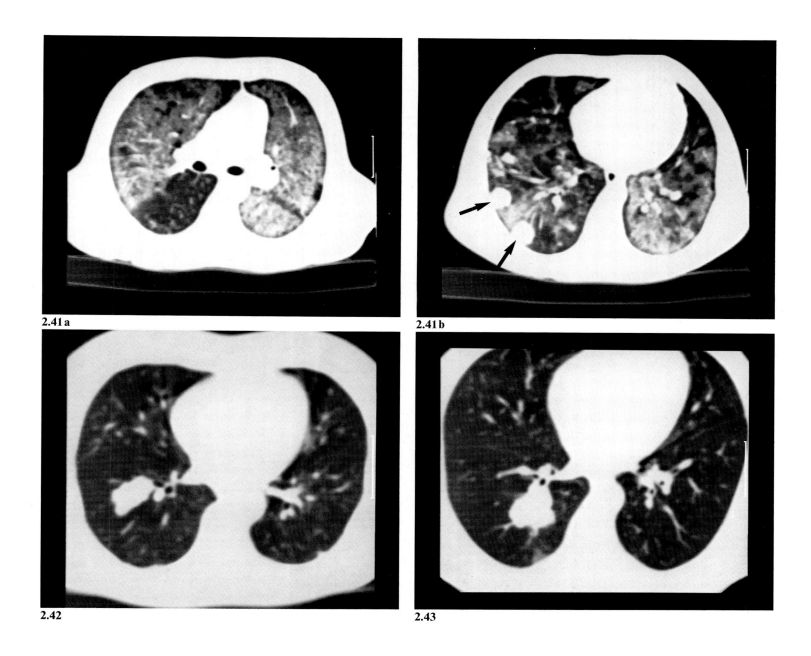

2.41 a   2.41 b

2.42   2.43

Fig. 2.41 a, b. Alveolar proteinosis. S 8 mm; WW 1024 HU; WL −600 HU. **a** Section through middle lung regions. **b** Section through lower lung regions.

Extensive coalescent consolidations are inhomogeneously spread over both lungs, sparing a small subpleural space. There are well-defined denser nodules in the right lower lobe (→)

Fig. 2.42. Bronchial adenoma, carcinoid type. S 4 mm; WW 1500 HU; WL −700 HU.

A homogeneous, sharply circumscribed and slightly lobulated mass arises from the lateral basal segmental bronchus of the right lower lobe. The tumour extends into the contiguous lung parenchyma but does not protrude into the bronchial lumen

Fig. 2.43. Peripheral oat cell bronchogenic carcinoma. S 4 mm; WW 1500 HU; WL −700 HU.

A lobulated mass extends from the posterior segmental bronchus of the right lower lobe and involves the surrounding lung parenchyma; no bronchial deformity can be seen. The malignant tumour is equivalent to the benign adenoma demonstrated in Fig. 2.42

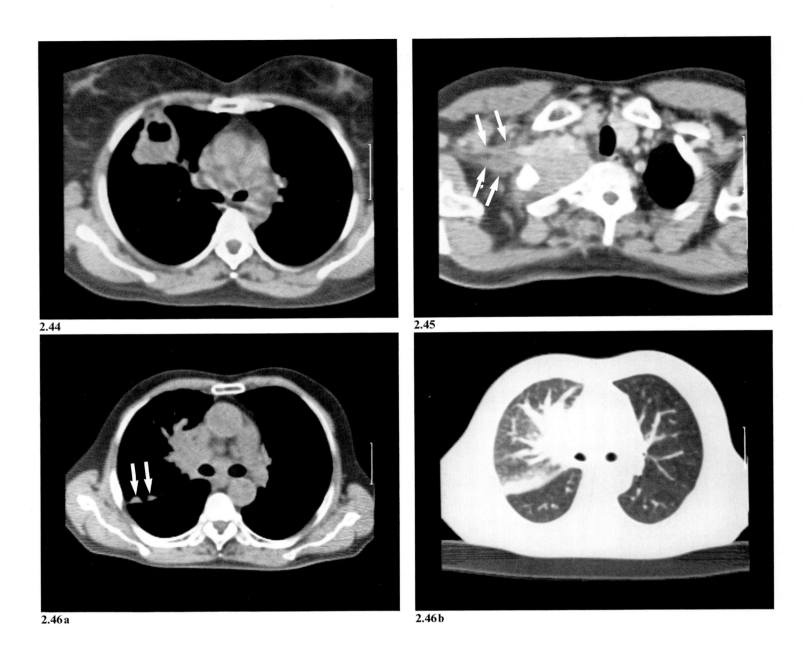

2.44

2.45

2.46 a

2.46 b

Fig. 2.44. Peripheral squamous cell bronchogenic carcinoma with cavitation. S 8 mm; WW 512 HU; WL +40 HU.

There is a sharply demarcated mass in the anterior segment of the right upper lobe with an irregularly shaped eccentric air-containing space and pleural involvement. Also shown are tracheobronchial lymph node metastases with stellar motion artefacts around the left main bronchus

Fig. 2.45. Pancoast tumour. S 8 mm; WW 512 HU; WL +40 HU.

This contrast-enhanced scan shows a right apical mass, which has infiltrated the right-sided subclavian vessels and the adjacent brachial plexus ($\rightarrow\rightarrow$)

Fig. 2.46a, b. Central oat cell bronchogenic carcinoma. **a** S 8 mm; WW 512 HU; WL +50 HU. **b** Same section; WW 1024 HU; WL −800 HU.

The scan shows a right hilar neoplasm with complete poststenotic atelectasis of the apical segment and hypoventilation of the remaining right upper lobe. Note the peripheral extension of the tumour with subpleural masses ($\rightarrow$) along the right oblique fissure; there are tracheobronchial lymph node metastases

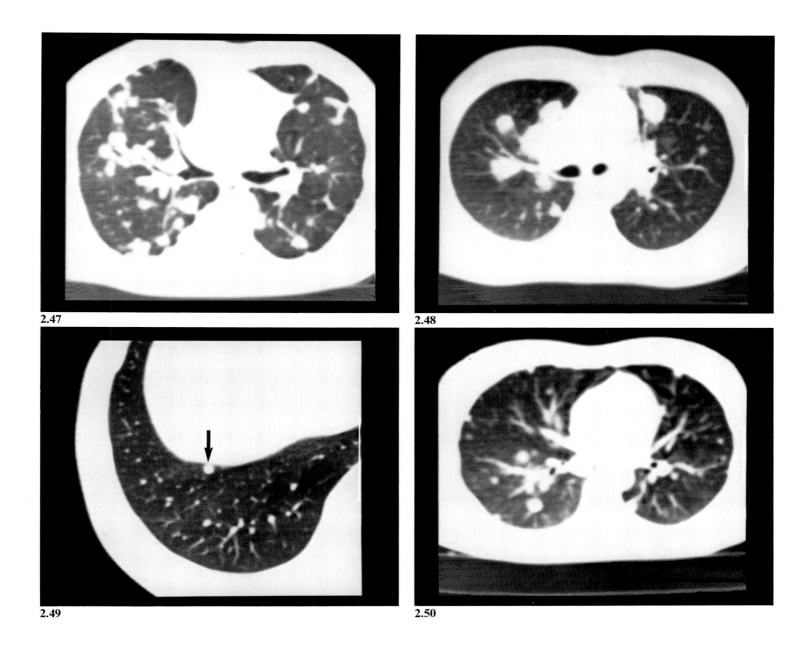

2.47

2.48

2.49

2.50

Fig. 2.47. Disseminated alveolar cell carcinoma. S 4 mm; WW 1500 HU; WL −750 HU.

Features shown are prominent line densities along the bronchovascular bundles; widely disseminated, more or less confluent nodules with irregular margins and thickenings of adjacent pleura regions in both lungs; and parenchymal shrinkages with forward displacement of the right posterior segmental bronchus

Fig. 2.48. Hodgkin's disease. S 8 mm; WW 1500 HU; WL −600 HU.

There is mediastinal and bilateral hilar lymph node involvement. Most of the multiple space-occupying consolidations in both lungs are distributed along central bronchovascular bundles

Fig. 2.49. Solitary pulmonary metastasis from synovialoma. Section zooming; S 2 mm; WW 1500 HU; WL −700 HU.

The small nodule in the right posterior phrenicocostal angle (→) could not be detected by conventional radiography. CT is more sensitive than conventional X-ray techniques in detecting small pulmonary nodules, especially when they are located in the peripheral subpleural spaces or in the phrenicocostal sinuses. By analysing CT values, intranodular calcifications can be identified at an earlier stage and well localized, bringing improved discrimination between benign and malignant nodules

Fig. 2.50. Multiple pulmonary metastases from malignant phaeochromocytoma. S 8 mm; WW 1024 HU; WL −800 HU

39

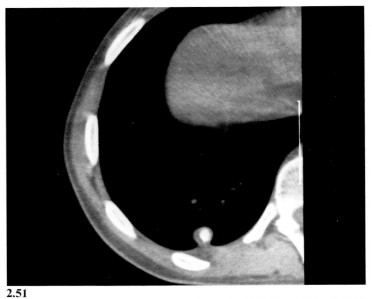

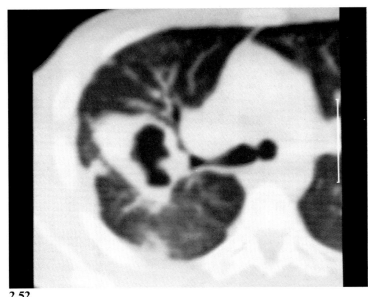

2.51

2.52

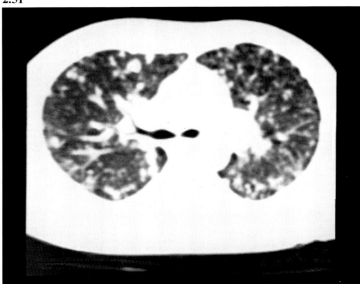

2.53

Fig. 2.51. Calcified pulmonary metastasis from osteogenic sarcoma. Section zooming; S 2 mm; WW 1024 HU; WL +50 HU.

The subpleural nodule displays eccentric calcification and pleural involvement

Fig. 2.53. Disseminated lymphangitic metastases from thyroid carcinoma. S 8 mm; WW 1024 HU; WL −800 HU.

Multiple nodules of different sizes are widely scattered throughout both lungs. There is accentuation of bronchovascular markings and bilateral hilar lymph node enlargement

Fig. 2.52. Cavitated pulmonary metastasis from testicular teratoma. Enlarged section; S 8 mm; WW 2046 HU; WL −700 HU.

There is a large space-occupying mass in the right upper lobe with an eccentric, irregularly shaped air-containing space. Note also thickening of the adjacent pleura, infiltrations in the superior segment of the right lower lobe and enlarged hilar lymph nodes

References

1. Adler O, Rosenberger A (1980) Computed tomography in guiding of fine needle aspiration biopsy of the lung and mediastinum. Fortschr Röntgenstr 133:135–137
1a. Aronberg DJ, Sagel SS (1981) High CT attenuation value of a benign pulmonary nodule. J Comput Assist Tomogr 5:563–564
2. Asai N (1979) Studies on the pleural space following pneumectomy (in Japanese). Nippon Kyobu Shikkan Gakkai Zasshi 17:476–482
3. Ayers WR, Huang HK (1979) The use of computerized tomography in the diagnosis of pulmonary nodules. Comput Tomogr 2:55–62
4. Baber CE, Hedlund LW, Oddson TA, Putman CE (1980) Differentiating empyemas and peripheral pulmonary abscesses: the value of computed tomography. Radiology 135:755–758
5. Berger PE, Kulu JP, Kuhns LR (1980) Computed tomography and the occult tracheobronchial foreign body. Radiology 134:133–135
6. Berger JL, Shaft MJ (1981) Pulmonary lymphangioleiomyomatosis. J Comput Assist Tomogr 5:565–576
7. Blane CE, Donn SM, Mori KW (1981) Congenital cystic adenomatoic malformation of the lung. J Comput Assist Tomogr 5:418–420
8. Bledin A, Bernardino ME, Libshitz HJ (1980) Cardiophrenic angle nodes: an unusual CT finding of advanced metastatic disease. CT 4:193–196
9. Brown LR, Muhm RM, Sheedy II PF (1981) Computed tomography of the chest. In: Putman CE (ed) Pulmonary diagnosis. Imaging and other techniques. Appleton Century Crofts, New York
10. Chang AE, Schaner EG, Conkle DM, Flye MW, Doppman JL, Rosenberg SA (1979) Evaluation of computed tomography in the detection of pulmonary metastases: a prospective study. Cancer 43:913–916
11. Chevalier PA, Wood EH, Robb RA, Ritman EL (1980) Synchronous volumetric computed tomography for quantitative studies of structural and functional dynamics of the respiratory system. In: Matthys H (ed) Progress in respiration research. Biomedical engineering and data processing in pneumonology. Karger, Basel
12. Creagan ET, Frytak S, Pairolero P, Hahn RG, Muhm JR (1979) Surgically proven pulmonary metastases not demonstrated by computed chest tomography. Cancer Treat Rep 62:1404–1405
13. Döhring W (1980) Quantitative analyses of regional pulmonary ventilation using Compton densitometry and computed tomography. In: Matthys H (ed) Progress in respiration research. Biomedical engineering and data processing in pneumonology. Karger, Basel
14. Döhring W, Linke G (1979) Die Grundlagen der quantitativen Computer-Tomographie. Fortschr Röntgenstr 130:133–143
15. Döhring W, Linke G (1979) Die Anwendung der Computer-Tomographie zur quantitativen Belüftungsanalyse der Lunge. Atemwegs- und Lungenkrankheiten 5:144–152
16. Döhring W, Linke G, Stender HS (1981) CT densitometry of the lung. In: Donner MW, Heuck FHW (eds) Radiology Today 1. Springer, Berlin Heidelberg New York
17. Ekholm SE, Albrechtson U, Kugelberg J, Tylén U (1980) Computed tomography in preoperative staging of bronchogenic carcinoma. J Comput Assist Tomogr 4:763–765
18. Emami B, Melo A, Carter BL, Munzenrider JE, Piro AJ (1978) Value of computed tomography in radiotherapy of lung cancer. Am J Roentgenol 131:63–67
19. Felix R, Wegener OH (1981) Computed tomography in space-occupying lesions in the thoracic area. Eur J Radiol 1:345–347
20. Foley WD, Lawson TL, Scanlon GT, Heeschen RC, Dibianca F (1979) Digital radiograph of the chest using a computed tomography instrument. Radiology 133:231–234
21. Fullerton GD, Sewchand W, Payne JT, Levitt SH (1978) CT determination of parameters for inhomogeneity corrections in radiation therapy of the esophagus. Radiology 126:167–171
22. Galluzzi S, Covielli G, Forzini L, Ferrari F, Stuart C (1980) Farmer's lung: comparison of the teleradiographic images and computerized tomographic (CT) images (in Italian). Radiol Med (Torino) 65:207–212
23. Godwin JD, Webb WR, Gamsu G, Ovenfors CO (1980) Computed tomography of pulmonary embolism. Am J Roentgenol 135:691–695
24. Grossman ZD, Thomas FD, Gagne G, Mauceri R, Cohen WN, Heitzman ER, Singh A (1979) Transmission computed tomographic diagnosis of experimentally produced acute pulmonary vascular occlusion in the dog. Radiology 131:767–769
25. Grossman ZD, Gagne G, Zens A, Thomas FD, Chamberlain CC, Singh A, Cohen WN, Heitzman ER (1980) Transmission computed tomography, Tc-99m MAA scintigraphy, and plain chest radiography after experimentally produced acute pulmonary arterial occlusion in the dog. J Nucl Med 20:1251–1256
26. Gur D, Drayer BP, Borovetz HS, Griffith BP, Hardesty RL, Wolfson SK (1979) Dynamic computed tomography of the lung: regional ventilation measurements. J Comput Assist Tomogr 3:749–753
27. Gur D, Shabason L, Borovitz HS, Hertert DL, Reece GJ, Kennedy WH, Serago C (1981) Regional pulmonary ventilation measurements by xenon enhanced dynamic computed tomography: an update. J Comput Assist Tomogr 5:678–683
28. Haage JR, Reich NE, Havrilla TR, Alfidi RJ (1978) Computed tomography—guided biopsy. CT 1:25–30
29. Haertel M, Fretz C, Fuchs WA (1980) Zur computertomographischen Diagnostik der Echinokokkose. Fortschr Roentgenstr 133:164–170
30. Haertel M, Tillmann U, Fuchs WA (1980) Thorakale Computer-Tomographie. Dtsch Med Wochenschr 104:1610–1612
31. Hedlund L, Friedman M, Effman E, Outman CE (1981) Lung density measurement by computed tomography. Am Rev Respir Dis 123:245
32. Hedlund LW, Putman CE (1981) Analysis of lung density by computed tomography. In: Putman CE (ed) Pulmonary diagnosis. Imaging and other techniques. Appleton Century Crofts, New York
33. Heitzman ER (1981) CT of the thorax. Am J Radiol 136:2–12
34. Heitzman ER, Proto AV, Goldwin RL (1979) The role of computerized tomography in the diagnosis of diseases of the thorax. JAMA 241:933–936
35. Husband JE, Peckham MJ, MacDonald JS, Hendry WF (1979) The role of computed tomography in the management of testicular teratoma. Clin Radiol 30:243–252
36. Isherwood J, Best JJK (1980) The use of computed tomography in lung disease. In: Flenley (ed) Recent advances in respiratory medicine. Churchill Livingstone, Edinburgh
37. Ishida I, Fukuma S, Sawada K, Seki Y, Tanaka F, Tanaka K (1980) Whole lung computed tomography for detection of pulmonary metastasis of osteosarcoma confirmed at thoracotomy (in Japanese). Nippon Kyobo Geka Gakkai Zasshi 28:60–67
38. Jost RG, Sagel SS, Stanley RJ, Levitt RG (1978) Computed tomography of the thorax. Radiology 126:125–136
39. Kagan AR, Steckel RJ, Bein ME, Holmes EC (1981) Pulmonary mass in a smoker: preoperative imaging for staging of lung cancer. Am J Radiol 136:739–745
40. Katz D, Kreel L (1979) Computed tomography in pulmonary asbestosis. Clin Radiol 30:207–213

41. Kawakami M, Abe S, Yamaguchi M, Konno K, Takizawa T (1979) Computer tomography of cryptogenic fibrosing alveolitis (in Japanese). Nippon Kyobu Shikkan Gakkai Zasshi 17:348–354

42. Keller MJ, Edwards FM, Rundle R (1981) Automatic outlining of regions on CT scans. J Comput Assist Tomogr 5:240–245

43. Kirks DR, Korobkin M (1980) Computed tomography for chest examinations in children. Pediatr Ann 9:192–199

44. Kollins SA (1978) Computed tomography of the pulmonary parenchyma and chest wall. Radiol Clin North Am 15:297–308

45. Kreel L (1976) Computer tomography in the evaluation of pulmonary asbestosis. Preliminary experiences with the EMI general purpose scanner. Acta Radiol [Diagn] (Stockh) 17:405–412

46. Kreel L (1977) The EMI body scanner. An interim clinical evaluation. J Neuroradiol 3:159–182

47. Kreel L (1978) Computed tomography of the lung and pleura. Semin Roentgenol 13:213–225

48. Kreel L (1979) Computer tomography of the thorax. Radiol Clin North Am 16:575–584

49. Kruglik GD, Wayne KS (1980) Occult lung cavity causing hemoptysis: recognition by computed tomography. J Comput Assist Tomogr 4:407–408

50. Kuckein D, Dobbelstein D (1980) Bochdaleksche Zwerchfellhernie – ein computertomographischer Beitrag zur roentgenologischen Differentialdiagnose eines intrapulmonalen Rundherdes dorsobasal. Fortschr Roentgenstr 131:327–328

51. Kuhns LR, Borlaza GS, Seigel RS (1979) Rapid sequence display of computed tomographic images: an aid in the diagnosis of pulmonary metastases. Radiology 132:747–748

52. Kuhns LR, Borlaza G (1980) The "twinkling star" sign: an aid in differentiating pulmonary vessels from pulmonary nodules on computed tomograms. Radiology 135:763–764

53. Kutzen B (1980) Computed tomography of the chest. J Maine Med Assoc 71:72–74

54. Lackner K, Bücheler E, Buurmann R, Felix R, Heuser L, Mödder U, Oeser H, Wegener OH (1979) Diagnostische Möglichkeiten der Computer-Tomographie im Thoraxbereich. Roentgenpraxis 31:229–232

55. Lackner K, Felix R, Oeser H, Wegener OH, Bücheler E, Buurmann R, Heuser L, Mödder U, Thurn P (1978) Erweiterung der Roentgendiagnostik im Thoraxbereich durch die Computer-Tomographie. Radiologe 19:79–89

56. Machida K, Itai Y, Yashiro N, Hurui S, Machida T, Yoshikawa H, Tasaka H (1979) Evaluation of radiographic CT diagnosis of the mediastinum and the lung (in Japanese). Nippon Rinsho 37:43–46

57. McCook TA, Kirks DR, Merten DE, Osborne DR, Spock A, Pratt PC (1981) Pulmonar alveolar proteinosis in children. Am J Radiol 137:1023–1027

58. McLoud TC, Wittenberg J, Ferrucci JT Jr (1979) Computed tomography of the thorax and standard radiographic evaluation of the chest: a comparative study. J Comput Assist Tomogr 3:170–180

59. Mintzer RA (1981) Chest imaging – an integrated approach. Williams & Wilkins, Baltimore

60. Mintzer RA, Malave SR, Neiman HL, Michaelis LL, Vanecko RM, Sanders JH (1979) Computed vs. conventional tomography in evaluation of primary and secondary pulmonary neoplasm. Radiology 132:653–659

61. Muhm JR (1980) Role of computed tomography in evaluation of intrathoracic lesions. J Thorac Cardiovasc Surg 79:469–470

62. Muhm JR, Brown LR, Crowe JK (1977) Detection of pulmonary nodules by computed tomography. Am J Roentgenol 128:267–270

63. Muhm JR, Brown LR, Crowe JK (1977) Use of computed tomography in the detection of pulmonary nodules. Mayo Clin Proc 52:345–348

64. Muhm JR, Brown LR, Crowe JK, Sheedy PF, Hattery RR, Stephens DH (1979) Comparison of whole lung tomography and computed tomography for detecting pulmonary nodules. Am J Roentgenol 131:981–984

65. Müller HA, Van Kaick G, Schaaf J, Lülling H, Vogt-Moykopf J, Delphendahl A (1981) Proäoperatives Staging des Bronchialcarcinoms: Wertigkeit der Computer-Tomographie im Vergleich zur konventionellen Radiologie. Fortschr Röntgenstr 134:601–607

66. Nabawi P, Mantrawadi R, Breyer D, Capetz V (1981) Computed tomography of radiation-induced lung injuries. J Comput Assist Tomogr 5:568–570

67. Nachman JB, Baum ES, White H, Cruissi FG (1981) Bleomycin-induced pulmonary fibrosis mimicking recurrent metastatic disease in a patient with testicular carcinoma: case report of CT scan appearance. Cancer 47:236–239

68. Naidich DP, Khouri NF, Scott WW Jr, Wang KP, Siegelman SS (1981) Computed tomography of the pulmonary hila: 1. normal anatomy. J Comput Assist Tomogr 5:459–467

69. Naidich DP, Khouri NF, Stitik FP, McCauley DJ, Siegelman SS (1981) Computed tomography of the pulmonary hila: 2. abnormal anatomy. J Comput Assist Tomogr 5:468–475

70. Naidich DP, Stitik FP, Khouri NF, Terry PB, Siegelman SS (1980) Computed tomography of the bronchi. 2. Pathology. J Comput Assist Tomogr 4:754–762

71. Naidich DP, Terry PB, Stitik FP, Siegelman SS (1980) Computed tomography of the bronchi. 1. Normal anatomy. J Comput Assist Tomogr 4:746–753

72. Paling MR, Dwyer A (1980) The first rib as the cause of a "pulmonary nodule" on the chest computed tomography. J Comput Assist Tomogr 4:847–848

73. Pugatch RD, Faling LJ, Robbins AH, Snider GL (1978) Differentiation of pleural and pulmonary lesions using computed tomography. J Comput Assist Tomogr 2:601–606

74. Raptopoulos V, Schellinger D, Katz S (1978) Computed tomography of solitary pulmonary nodules: experience with scanning times longer than breath-holding. J Comput Assist Tomogr 2:55–60

75. Raval B, Ahmad D, Mathur P (1979) Alveolar cell carcinoma on CT scanning. The value of the air bronchogram sign. J Can Assoc Radiol 30:64–65

76. Ritman EL, Robb RA, Johnson SA, Chevalier PA, Gilbert BK, Greenleaf JF, Sturm RE, Wood EH (1978) Quantitative imaging of the structure and function of the heart, lungs, and circulation. Mayo Clin Proc 53:3–11

77. Robbins AH, Pugatch RD, Gerzof SG, Faling LJ, Johnson WC, Sewell DH (1978) Observations on the medical efficiency of computed tomography of the chest and abdomen. Am J Roentgenol 131:15–19

78. Robinson PJ, Kreel L (1979) Pulmonary tissue attenuation with computed tomography: comparison of inspiration and expiration scans. J Comput Assist Tomogr 3:740–748

79. Rosenblum LJ, Mauceri RA, Wellenstein DE, Bassano DA, Cohen WN, Heitzman ER (1979) Computed tomography of the lung. Radiology 129:521–524

80. Rosenblum LJ, Mauceri RA, Wellenstein DE, Thomas FD, Bassano DA, Raasch BN, Chamberlain CC, Heitzman ER (1980) Density patterns in the normal lung as determined by computed tomography. Radiology 137:409–416

81. Rothman SL, Jaffe CC, Simeone JF (1980) Computerized tomography in the assessment of diseases of the thorax: a critical review. CRC Crit Rev Diagn Imaging 11:57–74

82. Sagel S, Stanley RJ, Evens RG (1976) Early clinical experience with motionless whole-body computed tomography. Radiology 119:321–330

83. Schaner EG, Chang AE, Doppman JL, Conkle DM, Flye MW, Rosenberg SA (1978) Comparison of computed and conventional whole lung tomography in detecting pulmonary nodules: a prospective radiologic-pathologic study. Am J Roentgenol 131:51–54

84. Schaner EG, Chang AE, Doppman JL, Conkle DM, Rosenberg SA (1977) Comparison of computed and conventional whole lung tomography in the detection of pulmonary metastases. J Comput Assist Tomogr 1:363

85. Schaner EG, Head GL, Kalman MA, Dunnick NR, Doppman JL (1978) Whole body computed tomography in the diagnosis of abdominal and thoracic malignancy: review of 600 cases. Cancer Treat Rep 61:1537–1560

86. Scheid KF, Lissner J, Blaha H, Gebauer A (1981) Densitometrische Analyse pulmonaler Rundherde im Computer-Tomogramm. Fortschr Röntgenstr 134:357–363

87. Scherer U (1977) Möglichkeiten der Computer-Tomographie in der Pneumonologie. Prax Klin Pneumol 31:381–383

88. Scholten ET, Kreel L (1977) Distribution of lung metastases in the axial plane. A combined radiological-pathological study. Radiol Clin (Basel) 46:248–265

89. Shevland JE, Chiu LC, Schapiro RL, Young JA, Rossi NP (1979) The role of conventional tomography and computed tomography in assessing the respectability of primary lung cancer: a preliminary report. CT 2:1–19

90. Siegelman SS (1979) Computed tomography. In: Siegelman SS, Stitik FP, Summer WR (eds) Pulmonary system: practical approaches to pulmonary diagnosis. Grune & Stratton, New York

91. Siegelman SS, Zerhouni EA, Leo FP, Khouri NF, Stitik FP (1980) CT of the pulmonary nodule. Am J Roentgenol 135:1–13

92. Sinner WN (1978) Computed tomographic patterns of pulmonary thromboembolism and infarction. J Comput Assist Tomogr 2:395–399

93. Sinner WN (1981) Computed tomography of "pleuroma"—a cancer-mimicking atelectatic pseudotumor of the lung. Eur J Radiol 1:266–269

94. Soila P (1978) Computed tomography (CT) in chest examinations. Scand J Respir Dis [Suppl] 102:181–183

95. Solomon A, Kreel L, McNicol M, Johnson N (1979) Computed tomography in pulmonary sarcoidosis. J Comput Assist Tomogr 3:754–758

96. Stiris MG, Brothwik R (1981) Computed tomography (CT) evaluation in pulmonary sarcoidosis. Eur J Radiol 1:16–19

97. Takayama M, Katsuyama N, Kawakami K, Tada S (1980) Comparison of computed tomography with radionuclide tomography in chest diagnosis (in Japanese). Kaku Igaku 16:695–705

98. Tsubota N, Ohyama T, Kubota H, Shirakawa M, Yoshie T, Okamoto M, Arao M (1980) Computed tomography of the chest in surgical case (in Japanese). Kyobu Geka 32:736–742

99. Underwood GH Jr, Hooper RG, Axelbaum SP, Goodwin DW (1979) Computed tomographic scanning of the thorax in the staging of bronchogenic carcinoma. N Engl Med J 300:777–778

100. Utell MJ, Wandtke JC, Fahey PJ, Baker A, Fischer HW, Hyde RW (1979) Lung weight in normal and edematous dogs by computerized tomography (abstr). Fed Proc 38:1326

101. Vock P, Haertel M (1981) Die Computer-Tomographie zur Stadieneinteilung des Bronchuscarcinoms. Fortschr Röntgenstr 134:131–135

102. Webb WR, Gamsu G, Glazer G (1981) Computed tomography of the abnormal pulmonary hilum. J Comput Assist Tomogr 5:485–490

103. Webb WR, Glazer G, Gamsu G (1981) Computed tomography of the normal pulmonary hilum. J Comput Assist Tomogr 5:476–484

104. Wegener OH (1979) Die Dichtebestimmung des Lungengewebes mittels Computer-Tomographie. Habilitationsschrift, Berlin

105. Wegener OH, Koeppe P, Oeser H (1978) Measurement of lung density by computed tomography. J Comput Assist Tomogr 2:263–273

106. Wegener OH, Koeppe P, Oeser H (1979) Lung density measurements by computed tomography. In: Gerhardt P, Van Kaick G (eds) Total body computerized tomography. Thieme, Stuttgart, pp 32–39

107. Williams TJ, Raval B, Ahmad D (1980) Progressive massive fibrosis developing after brief coal dust exposure: evaluation with CT scanning and radionuclide angiocardiography. JOM 22:21–24

108. Wright PH, Hanson A, Kreel L, Capel LH (1980) Respiratory function changes after asbestosis pleurisy. Thorax 35:31–36

109. Zaunbauer W, Robotti GC, Probst P, Haertel M, Schöpf R (1981) Zur Computer-Tomographie der Lungenaplasie. Fortschr Röntgenstr 135:682–685

CHAPTER 3

Pleura
and Thoracic Wall

P. VOCK and W.A. FUCHS

3.1 Introduction

Computer tomography conclusively demonstrates the topographical anatomy of both the thoracic wall and the adjacent pleura, thus closing the diagnostic gap between the superficial areas, accessible to clinical investigation, and the lungs, which are displayed to good advantage on conventional radiographs.

Based upon current experience, the following applications for CT of the pleura and thoracic wall are indicated:

Display of transverse topographical anatomy of soft tissue structures

Demonstration of minor pleural lesions, particularly within the costodiaphragmatic and paramediastinal areas

Detection of parietal inflammatory and neoplastic mass lesions

Staging of tumour invasion across anatomical borders

Evaluation of complex sequels of trauma.

3.2 Normal CT Anatomy of Thoracic Inlet

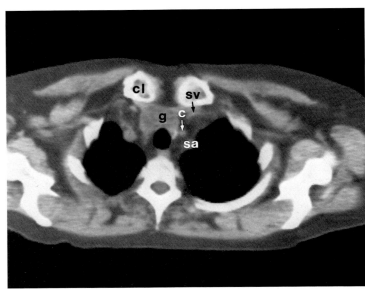

3.1 a

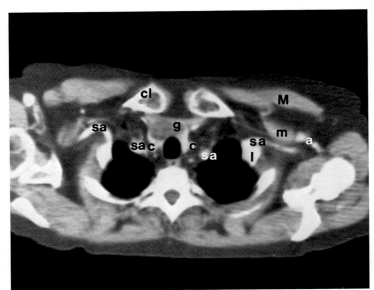

3.1 b

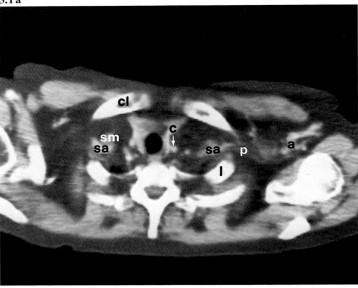

3.1 c

Fig. 3.1 a–c. Caudocranial sequence of scans with elevated arms. **a** Without contrast material. **b, c** After right brachial intravenous injection of contrast material. The subclavian vein (*sv*) courses ventrally and inferiorly from the mediastinum to the axilla; the subclavian artery (*sa*) and the brachial plexus (*p*) are identified dorsal to the scalenus anterior muscle (*sm*). Other structures are clearly visualized: clavicle (*cl*), first rib (*l*), minor (*m*) and major (*M*) pectoralis muscles, common carotid artery (*c*), axillary vessels (*a*), nodular goitre (*g*).

CT is superior to conventional radiography in the demonstration of soft tissue and osseous components of the thoracic inlet. Catheter angiography is preferable for the demonstration of vascular anatomy. Conventional radiography provides an overall view in the longitudinal plane (26)

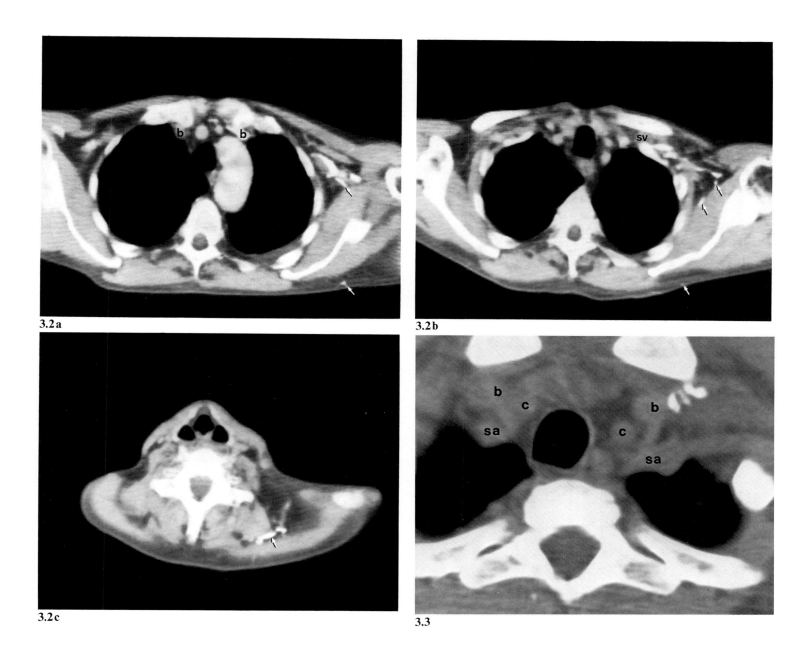

3.2a

3.2b

3.2c

3.3

Fig. 3.2a–c. Left subclavian vein thrombosis. Contrast-enhanced scans in caudocranial direction show soft tissue swelling and irregular interruption of contrast column within the subclavian vein (*sv*). Collaterals are demonstrated in the left axilla, the dorsal thoracic wall and the neck (*arrows*). Brachiocephalic veins (*b*) and arteries are patent and well filled with contrast medium.

CT demonstrates concomitant soft tissue inflammatory changes and vascular collaterals, rather than the exact morphology of venous thrombosis

Fig. 3.3 Localization of subclavian catheter fragments. Radiodense foreign bodies are identified outside the left brachiocephalic vein (*b*). The subclavian (*sa*) and common carotid (*c*) arteries are also demonstrated

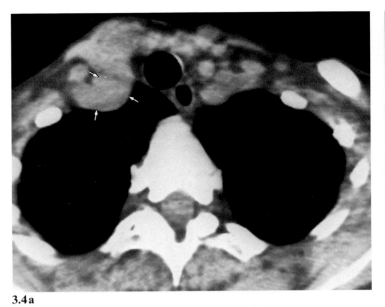

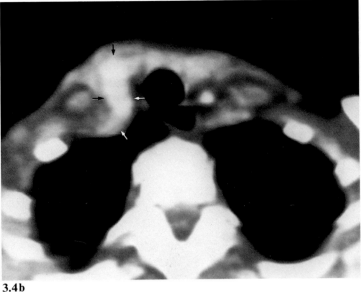

3.4a

3.4b

Fig. 3.4a, b. Ectasia of brachiocephalic trunk and right subclavian artery. Plain scan (**a**) and contrast-enhanced scan (**b**) showing the clinically palpable pulsating mass to be of vascular origin.

In selected cases CT provides conclusive diagnosis of vascular lesions of the thoracic wall, thus making catheter angiography unnecessary

3.4 Inflammatory Lesions

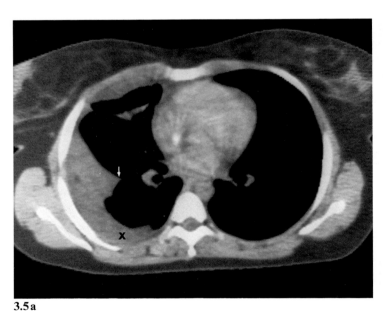

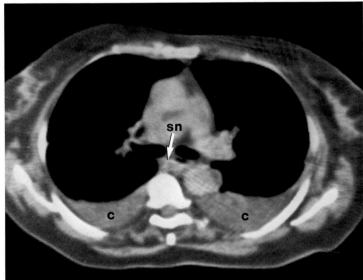

3.5a

3.5b

Fig. 3.5a. Pleural effusion (inflammatory). In the supine position, due to gravity, local pressure and surface tension, free pleural effusion is collected between the pleural surfaces dorsally (*x*), laterally and in the interlobar fissure (*arrow*), as a homogeneous crescent-shaped mass of low density (19 HU).

CT is very sensitive in detecting small quantities of pleural fluid (30 ml minimum) localized at first within the dorsal aspect of the pleural cavity [6, 9], enabling guided diagnostic or therapeutic puncture even when the fluid collection is loculated [7] (Fig. 3.15)

Fig. 3.5b. Chylothorax. There is a homogeneous collection of very low density (4 HU) caused by chylous effusion (*c*) in a patient with malignant non-Hodgkin's lymphoma (*sn*, subcarinal nodes).

The density of pleural fluid, depending on cellular, protein, lipid and haemoglobin content, sometimes distorted by cardiac motion artefacts, is of relative value in analysing the composition. Except in chylothorax (near 0 HU) and acute haemothorax (more than 40 HU; Fig. 3.9), there is a wide overlapping density range for transudation and infectious, neoplastic and other types of exudation [6]

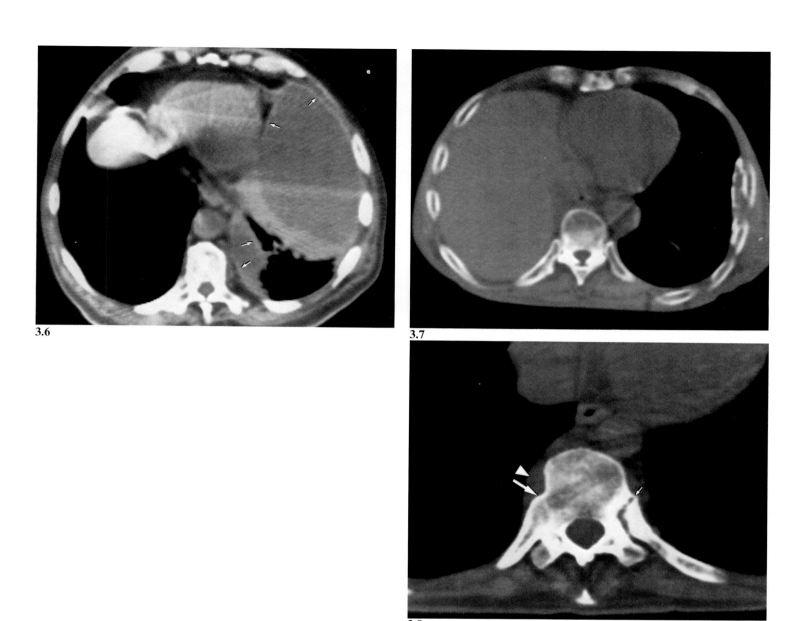

3.6

3.7

3.8

Fig. 3.6. Pleural empyema. Loculated purulent homogeneous exudate is seen in the left pleural cavity, and there is capsulation (*arrows*).

CT morphology of empyema depends on the stage of the disease [1, 6] with changing radiodensity according to maturation and organization. The diagnosis of empyema is made in correlation with clinical examination, unless gas accumulation due to anaerobic infection is present. Circumferential contrast enhancement due to inflammatory hyperaemia may be present. Empyema must be differentiated from lung abscess [2, 6, 21]. Phlegmonous infections and abscesses of the thoracic wall are well delineated

Fig. 3.7. Pleural scarring. Localized fibrotic calcified pleural thickening is a frequent residue of tuberculous pleurisy [6, 9]

Fig. 3.8. Costovertebral ankylosis in ankylosing spondylitis. Ossification of the costovertebral ligaments (*small arrow*) and ankylosis (*large arrow*) is accompanied by paravertebral soft tissue thickening (*arrowhead*).

CT demonstrates soft tissue components and osteoarticular alteration in ankylosing spondylitis

49

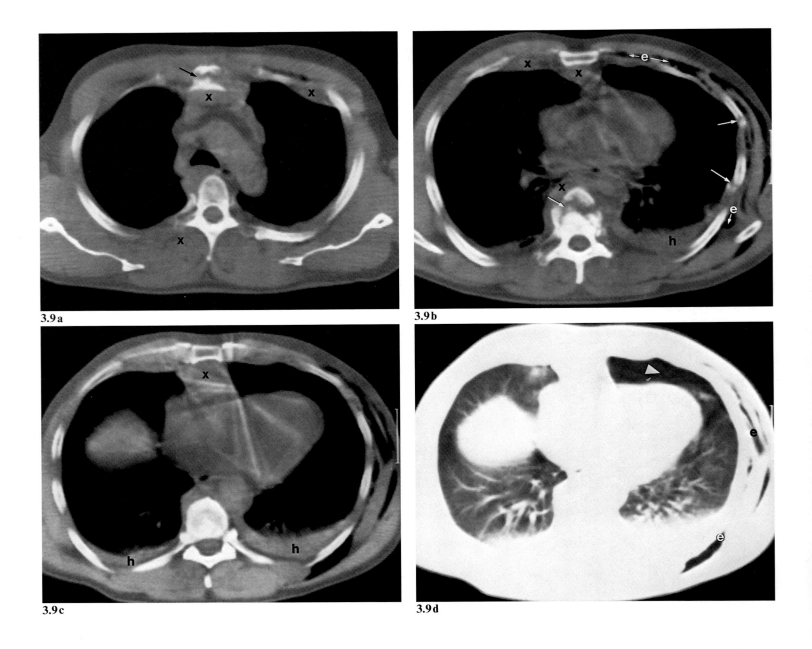

3.9a

3.9b

3.9c

3.9d

Fig. 3.9a–d. Multiple traumatic lesions to pleura and thoracic wall. **a** At T4 level; **b** at T7; **c** at T9; **d** at T9 with pulmonary window setting.

The patient presents fractures (*arrows*) of several ribs, spine and sternum, mediastinal and extrapleural parietal haematoma (*x*), bilateral haemothorax (*h*), left small ventral pneumothorax (*arrowhead*), lung disease (contusion) and thoracic wall emphysema (*e*) expanding along the muscle fascia.

CT visualizes in great detail the osseous, soft tissue and pulmonary extension of traumatic leions [21, 25]. However, conventional radiography is still the primary method for identification of traumatic lesions

3.6 Benign Neoplasm

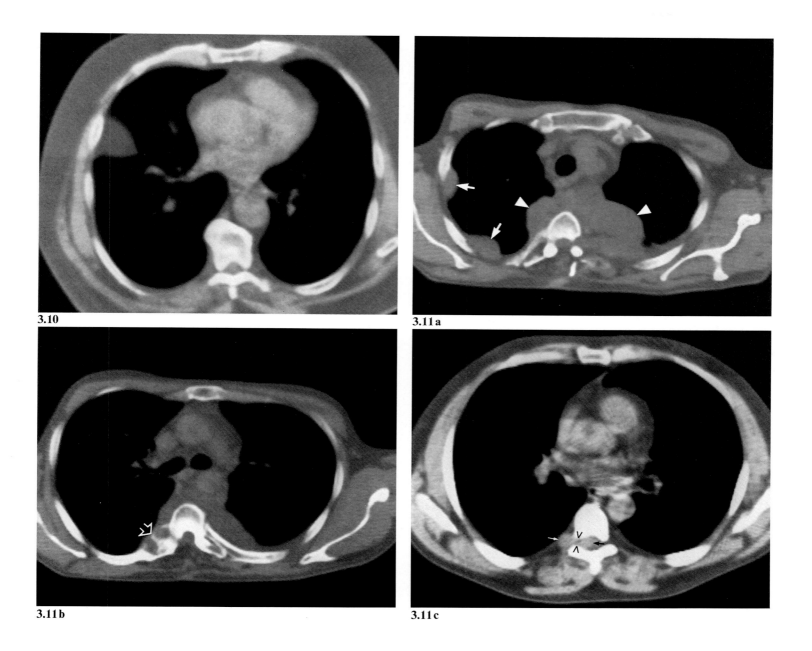

3.10

3.11 a

3.11 b

3.11 c

Fig. 3.10. Lipoma. This peripheral mass lesion contiguous to the right visceral pleural layer is characterized by a sharp borderline and a homogeneous radiodensity of −110 HU.

If partial volume effect can be excluded, CT density measurement allows the specific diagnosis of a thoracic lipoma and makes biopsy unnecessary. However, higher density values of −20 HU to −50 HU necessitate biopsy to exclude liposarcoma [14, 21]

Fig. 3.11 a–c. Neurofibromatosis and neurinoma [3, 8, 18]. **a** Multiple tumours arising from the intercostal nerves in close association with the inferior margin of the ribs (*arrows*) or from the spinal nerves (*arrowheads*). **b** Some are eroding vertebrae and ribs (*open arrow*). **c** Solitary neurinoma of hourglass shape (*arrows*) expanding through the intervertebral foramen (*black arrowheads*)

3.7 Primary Malignant Neoplasm

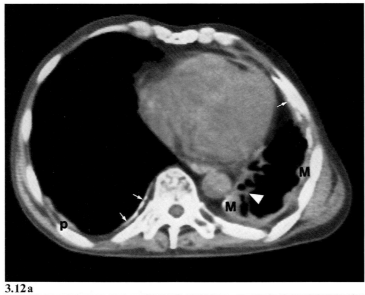

3.12 a

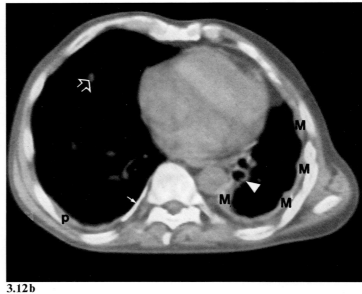

3.12 b

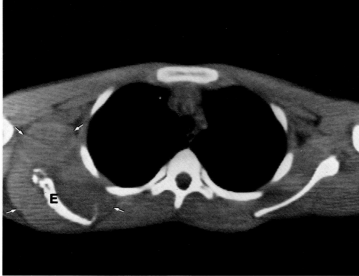

3.13

Fig. 3.12 a–b. Malignant pleural mesothelioma. The known occupational exposure and the fine bilateral pleural calcifications (*arrows*) and plaques (*p*) suggest asbestosis [9, 11, 12, 21]. Volume loss of the left hemithorax is caused by an irregular multilocular pleural tumour mass (*M*). The disease is in an advanced stage with infiltration of the left lung (*arrowhead*) and thoracic wall as well as haematogenous metastatic spread to the right lung (*open arrow*).

CT greatly facilitates the diagnosis of mesothelioma and conclusively evaluates the entire extension of the disease, providing valuable information even when there is additional pleural effusion or malignant infiltration through the diaphragm to the retroperitoneal and peritoneal space [6, 8, 9, 15, 22, 23]

Fig. 3.13. Ewing sarcoma of the right scapula. There is expansion and destruction of bone (*E*) with periosteal reaction at the medial margin and soft tissue infiltration to the infraspinatus, subscapularis and serratus anterior muscles (*arrows*)

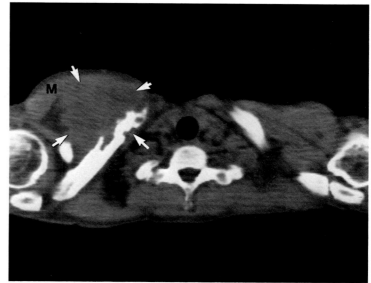

3.14a

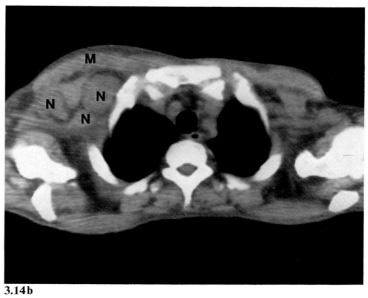

3.14b

Fig. 3.14a–b. Soft tissue sarcoma. **a** Right supraclavicular primary mass lesion (*arrows*), behind right pectoralis major muscle (*M*) and infiltrating the clavicle. **b** Infraclavicular and axillary lymph node metastases (*N*)

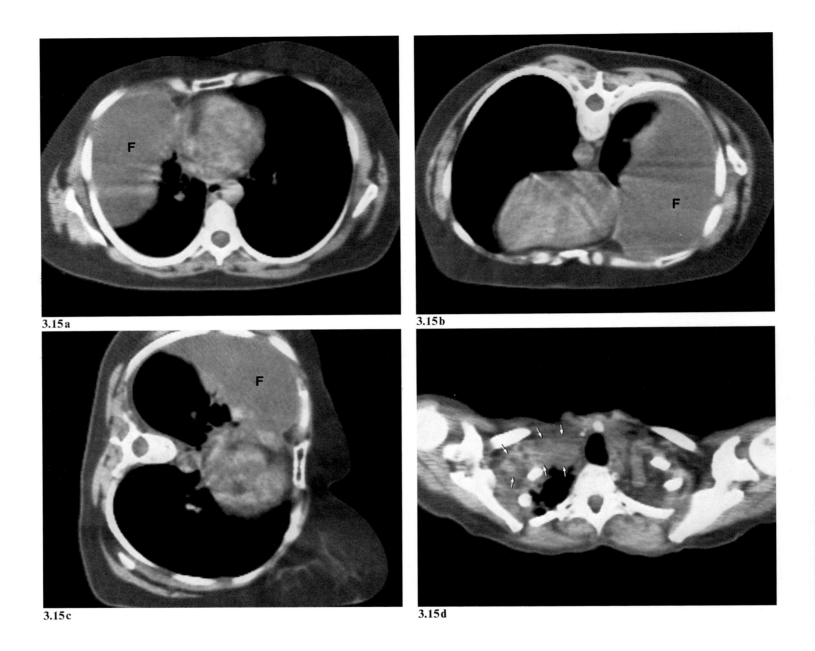

Fig. 3.15a–d. Carcinoma of the breast. Extension to pleura and thoracic inlet. The loculated pleural fluid (*F*) (12 HU), proved to be malignant by aspiration cytology, does not move in supine (**a**), prone (**b**) and left decubitus (**c**) positions. **d** Infiltration of right brachial nervous plexus (*arrows*) in another case of breast carcinoma with lymph node metastases.

CT may demonstrate or exclude space-occupying lesions, such as traumatic haematoma or tumour extension in breast cancer or Pancoast bronchogenic carcinoma [6, 26], as a cause of damage to the brachial nervous plexus

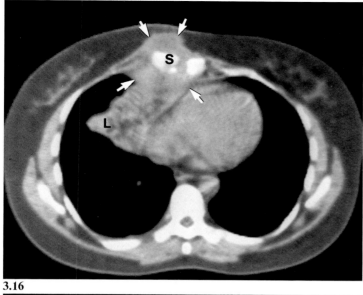

3.16

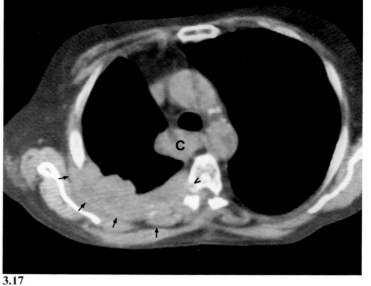

3.17

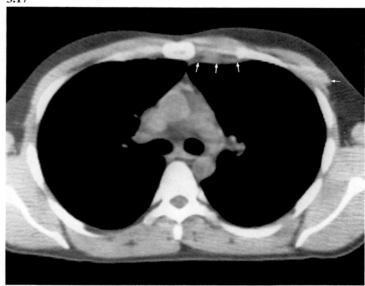

3.18a

3.18b

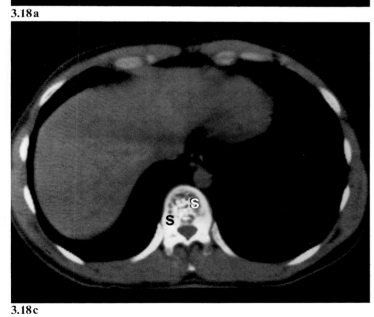

3.18c

Fig. 3.16. Hodgkin's disease. The lymphoma arises from the mediastinum and is locally invading sternal bone (*S*), peristernal soft tissues (*arrows*) and the middle lobe of the lung (*L*)

Fig. 3.17. Bronchogenic carcinoma. The pleuroparietal mass lesion (*C*) was disclosed 1 year after right bilobectomy. A dorsal mass infiltrates the vertebral body (*V*), transgressing the thoracic cage but respecting the fascial and fatty plane close to the subscapularis muscle (*arrows*).

Local thoracic wall invasion frequently occurs in Hodgkin's lymphoma [4, 8, 20] and bronchogenic carcinoma [19] and sometimes in pulmonary metastases [8]

Fig. 3.18a–c. Hodgkin's disease. CT clearly demonstrates left axillary (*A*) and mediastinal (*M*) lymph node enlargement, thoracic wall manifestations (*arrows*) and a sclerotic lesion of a lower dorsal vertebra (*S*).

Primary malignant lymphoma is frequently not limited to lymph nodes. CT is superior to conventional methods in demonstrating extranodular tumour localization [4, 17, 20]

3.9 Metastatic Disease

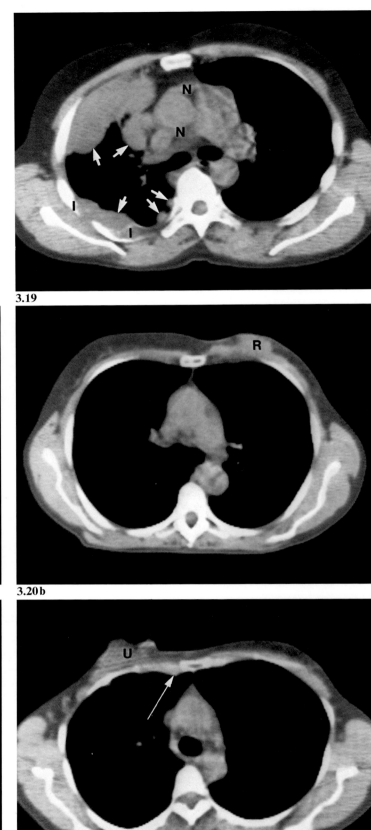

3.19

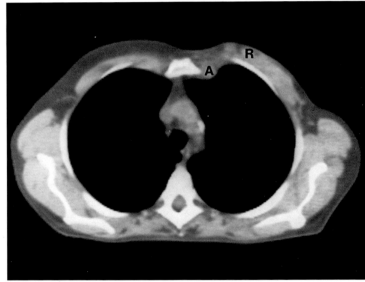

3.20 a

3.20 b

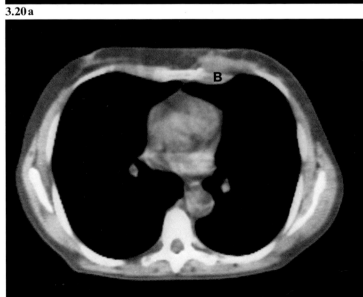

3.20 c

3.20 d

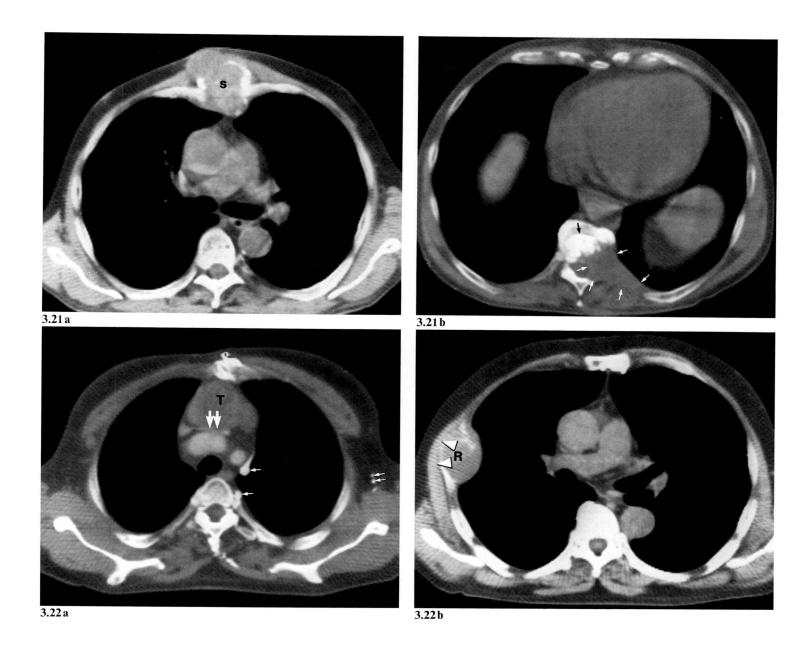

3.21 a

3.21 b

3.22 a

3.22 b

◁ **Fig. 3.19.** Pleural metastatic deposits of a malignant testicular tumour. The scan shows malignant pleural seeding (*arrows*) after right inferior lobectomy for solitary lung metastases, accompanied by secondary infiltration of ribs (*I*) and enlarged mediastinal lymph nodes (*N*)

◁ **Fig. 3.20 a–d.** Internal thoracic lymph node metastases of breast cancer. **a–c** Craniocaudal sequence of scans: local relapse of the primary tumour (*R*) infiltrating the thoracic wall. Malignant metastases involve the left internal thoracic (internal mammary) lymph nodes (*A, B*). **d** Ulcerating breast cancer (T4 stage; *U*) and enlarged right internal thoracic lymph node chain (*arrow*).

About 50% of patients with positive axillary nodes and tumours located in the central or inner portion of the breast have internal thoracic node involvement at the time of mastectomy [16]. Enlarged nodes of this chain are demonstrated by CT [24]

Fig. 3.21 a, b. Multiple myeloma. Localized destructive and partially sclerotic bone lesions of the sternum, with calcified soft tissue expansion (*S*), of vertebra T 10 and of the left tenth rib (*arrows*)

Fig. 3.22 a, b. Thyroid carcinoma. **a** Intrathoracic recurrence of thyroid cancer (*T*) with compression of the left brachiocephalic vein (*double arrow*) and collateral venous flow (*arrows*). **b** Haematogenous rib metastasis (*R*) causing an expansive extrapleural mass lesion and displacement of serratus anterior muscle (*arrowheads*).

CT demonstrates neoplastic lesions of the thoracic wall in their entirety, closing the diagnostic gap between superficial areas, accessible to clinical investigation, and the lungs, displayed on conventional radiographs [6, 7, 21]

References

1. Alexander JC Jr, Wolfe WG (1980) Lung abscess and empyema of the thorax. Surg Clin North Am 60:835–849
2. Baber CE, Hedlund LW, Oddson TA, Putman CE (1980) Differentiating empyemas and peripheral pulmonary abscess: the value of computed tomography. Radiology 135:755–758
3. Fraser RG, Paré JAP (1979) Diagnosis of diseases of the chest, vol III. WB Saunders, Philadelphia
4. Gouliamos AD, Carter BL, Emami B (1980) Computed tomography of the chest wall. Radiology 134:433–436
5. Haertel M, Tillmann U, Fuchs WA (1979) Thorakale Computertomographie. Dtsch Med Wochenschr 104:1610–1612
6. Hübener KH (1981) Computertomographie des Körperstammes. Thieme, Stuttgart
7. Kollins SA (1977) Computed tomography of the pulmonary parenchyma and chest wall. Radiol Clin North Am 15:297–308
8. Kreel L (1978) Computed tomography of the thorax. Radiol Clin North Am 16:575–584
9. Kreel L (1978) Computed tomography of the lung and pleura. Semin Roentgenol 13:213–225
10. Kreel L (1976) Computer tomography in the evaluation of pulmonary asbestosis. Acta Radiol Diagn 17:405–412
11. Kreel L (1979) Computed tomography in pulmonary asbestosis. Clin Radiol 30:207–213
12. Lackner K, Felix R, Oeser H, Wegener OH, Bücheler E, Buurman R, Heuser L, Mödder U, Thurn P (1979) Erweiterung der Röntgendiagnostik im Thoraxbereich durch die Computer-Tomographie. Radiologe 19:79–89
13. Lackner K, Brecht G, Janson R, Scherholz K, Lützeler A, Thurn P (1980) Wertigkeit der Computertomographie bei der Stadieneinteilung primärer Lymphknotenneoplasien. Fortschr Röntgenstr 132:21–30
14. Mendez G Jr, Isikoff MB, Isikoff SK, Sinner WN (1979) Fatty tumors of the thorax demonstrated by computerized tomography. AJR 133:207–212
15. Mischler NE, Chuprevich T, Johnson RO, Tormey DC (1979) Malignant mesothelioma presenting in the pleura and peritoneum. J Surg Oncol 11:185–191
16. Munzenrider JE, Tchakarova I, Castro M, Castro B (1979) Computerized body tomography in breast cancer. I. Internal mammary nodes and radiation treatment planning. Cancer 43:137–150
17. Pilepich MV, Rene JB, Munzenrider JE, Carter BL (1978) Contribution of computed tomography to the treatment of lymphomas. AJR 131:69–73
18. Stelzer P, Gay WA Jr (1980) Tumors of the chest wall. Surg Clin North Am 60:779–791
19. Vock P, Haertel M (1981) Die Computertomographie zur Stadieneinteilung des Bronchuskarzinoms. Fortschr Röntgenstr 134:131–135
20. Vock P, Haertel M, Fuchs WA (1981) Die thorakale Computertomographie beim Lymphoma malignum Hodgkin. Computertomographie 1:68–73
21. Van Moore A, Putman CE (1980) Radiologic diagnosis of chest disease. Surg Clin North Am 60:715–742
22. Alexander E, Clark RA, Colley DP, Mitchell SE (1981) CT of malignant pleural mesothelioma. AJR 137:287–291
23. Caron-Poitreau C, Delumeau J, Dabouis G, Petitier H, Rieux D (1981) Apport de la tomodensitométrie à l'étude des tumeurs primitives de la plèvre. Ann Radiol 24:247–253
24. Meyer JE, Munzenrider JE (1981) Computed tomographic demonstration of internal mammary lymph-node metastasis in patients with locally recurrent breast carcinoma. Radiology 139:661–663
25. Toombs BD, Sandler CM, Lester RG (1981) Computed tomography of chest trauma. Radiology 140:733–738
26. Webb WR, Jeffrey RB, Godwin JD (1981) Thoracic computed tomography in superior sulcus tumors. J Comput Assist Tomogr 5:361–365

CHAPTER 4

Mediastinum

A.L. Baert, P. Biondetti, T. Darras, P. De Somer,
L. Divano, J. Ferrané, A. Grivegnee, H. Hauser,
L. Jeanmart, D. Larde, M. Nijssens, M. Osteaux,
and N. Vasile

4.1 Normal Anatomy

L. Divano, M. Osteaux, and L. Jeanmart

The first "total body" CT scanners to be introduced into clinical work (in 1976) had only limited value in demonstrating the mediastinal structures, chiefly because their high scanning times permitted respiratory movements to have an adverse effect on spatial and densitometric resolution. The present systems, characterized by a pure rotary movement of the detection system and X-ray tube and by a great number of detectors, have seen a reduction in scanning time to 2–5 s. When suitable slice thicknesses and data processing programs are selected, the images obtained with voluntary apnoea provide a very accurate anatomical definition of mediastinal elements. However, further reductions in scanning time will be necessary to eliminate the impairment in depiction of vascular structures caused by cardiac movement.

In the present work, structures have been identified and "indexed" on the basis of our knowledge gained from classical books on anatomy and our own experience with anatomical investigation and in vivo selective opacification of the oesophagus and blood vessels. The principle to which we have adhered is simple: to present, side by side, two identical scans with optimal spatial resolution, and to identify as many of the structures as possible on one of these scans.

The CT system used was a Somatom S.F. scanner (Siemens AG). In order to improve spatial resolution, images were realized (slice thickness, 4 mm) and reconstructed in direct enlargement, starting from raw data ("zooming").

The images printed come from examinations performed within the framework of systematic screening or follow-up examinations of patients with extrathoracic malignant haemopathies in whom the existence of normal mediastinal structures was subsequently established. Vascular structures were, if necessary, studied after intravenous opacification by rapid i.v. injection of 50 cc Telebrix 38 with series of images every 11 s. These structures are sometimes confused with an "added" pathological picture on account of a frequent lack of symmetry in this area.

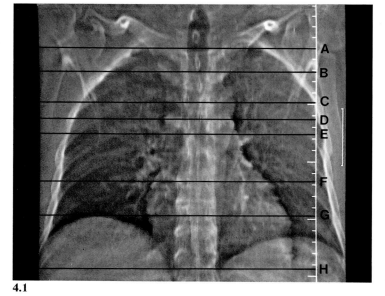

4.1

Fig. 4.1. Systematization of slice levels. On the basis of clinical interest, which centres upon primitive tumoral lesions and adenopathies, eight levels are to be distinguished:

A Cervicothoracic inlet
B Superior mediastinal (supra-aortic)
C Aortic arch
D Aortopulmonary window
E Tracheal bifurcation
F Left atrial
G Left ventricular
H Inferoposterior mediastinal

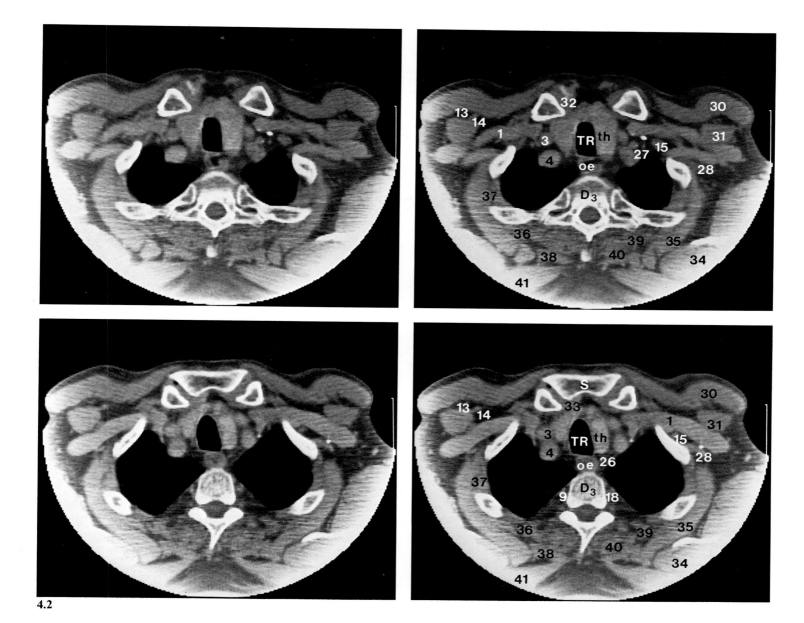

Fig. 4.2. Cervicothoracic inlet level. The scan is tangential to the upper border of the lungs (level T 2–T 3) and beyond or at the same height as the upper extremity of the manubrium sterni. The lower part of the lobes of the thyroid gland, with a high-density significant iodine content, encloses the trachea. The thyroïd is encircled by the carotid and subclavian arteries, whereas the venous element (brachiocephalic trunks) reaches the mediastinum from the axillary area. Behind the sternal manubrium, an adjacent opacity corresponds to the sternohyoïdian and sternothyroïdian muscles

1	Subclavian vein
3	Right carotid artery
4	Subclavian artery
9	Right superior intercostal vein
13	Suprascapular artery
14	Suprascapular vein
15	Internal thoracic artery

18	Intercostal vein
26	Laryngeal, recurrent nerve
27	Phenic nerve
28	Brachial plexus
30	Pectoralis major muscle
31	Pectoralis minor muscle
33	Sternohyoïdian and sternothyroidian muscle
34	Subscapularis muscle
35	Teres major muscle
36	Teres minor muscle
37	Intercostal muscle
38	Rhomboid major muscle
39	Longissimus thoracis muscle
40	Transversospinalis muscle
41	Trapezius muscle
TR	Trachea
oe	Oesophagus
S	Sternum

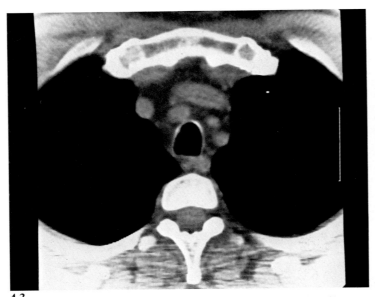

4.3

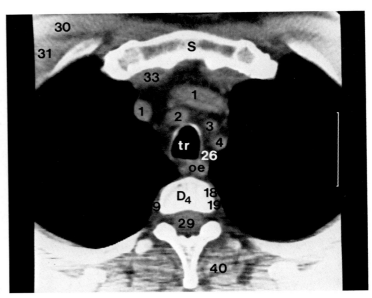

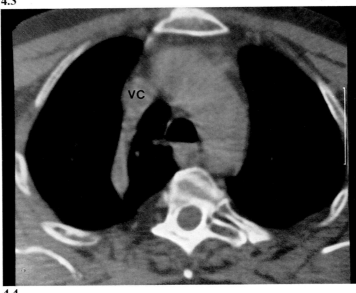

4.4

Fig. 4.3. Superior mediastinal (supra-aortic) level. The scan is at the level of T 4, at the same height as the manubrium sterni. The mediastinum appears here as a triangle with a round apex. No contrast medium is needed to identify with ease (a) the posterior sternal muscles; (b) the venous structures (brachiocephalic trunks); and (c) the brachiocephalic, carotid and subclavian arteries. These structures lie in a semicircle, from front to back. The oesophagus (here empty) appears as a small opacity on the left posterior face of the trachea. The lymph nodes of the area are small and poorly identified. In favourable cases (cooperative patient, sufficient mediastinal fat), the recurrent nerves are visualized in the immediate neighbourhood of the trachea

1   Brachiocephalic vein
2   Brachiocephalic artery
3   Left carotid artery
4   Subclavian artery

9   Right superior intercostal vein
18   Intercostal vein
19   Intercostal artery
26   Recurrent laryngeal nerve
29   Spinal cord
30   Pectoralis major muscle
31   Pectoralis minor muscle
33   Sternohyoidian and sternothyroidian muscle
40   Transversospinalis muscle
tr   Trachea
oe   Oesophagus
S   Sternum

Fig. 4.4. Azygos lobe. The azygos arch makes its way through the pleural reflection to the vena cava (*vc*)

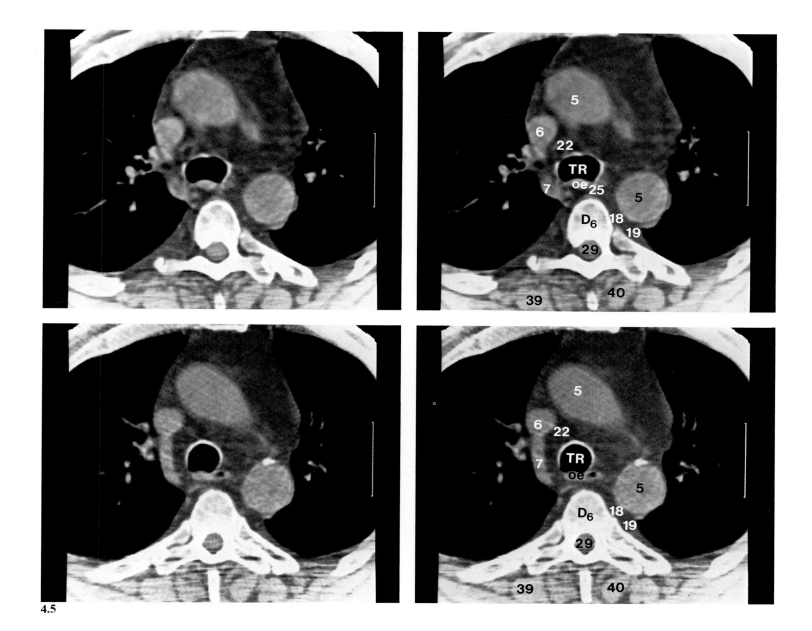

Fig. 4.5. Aortopulmonary window level. These scans at the height of T 6 also show the azygos arch and its junction with the vena cava. In and above the azygos arch, the inferior part of the Barety space is to be found; at this level some thin round opacities corresponding to normal lymph nodes can be seen.

The aortopulmonary window space, which contains the left pretracheobronchial chain lymph nodes, is bordered at the top, front and back by the aorta, inside by the trachea, outside by the pleura and below by hilary structures. It is to be noted that the pleural reflection limiting this space is concave towards the outside and that the azygos vein is first seen lateral and to the right of the oesophagus. The border of the oesophagus is not to be distinguished from the trachea, which is anterior to it. On the other hand, there is an obvious fatty interface between the oesophagus and the posterior osseous plane and aorta

5	Aorta
6	Superior vena cava
7	Azygos vein
18	Intercostal vein
19	Intercostal artery
22	Right tracheobronchial lymph node group
25	Thoracic duct
29	Spinal cord
39	Longissimus thoracis muscle
40	Transversospinalis muscle
TR	Trachea
oe	Oesophagus

63

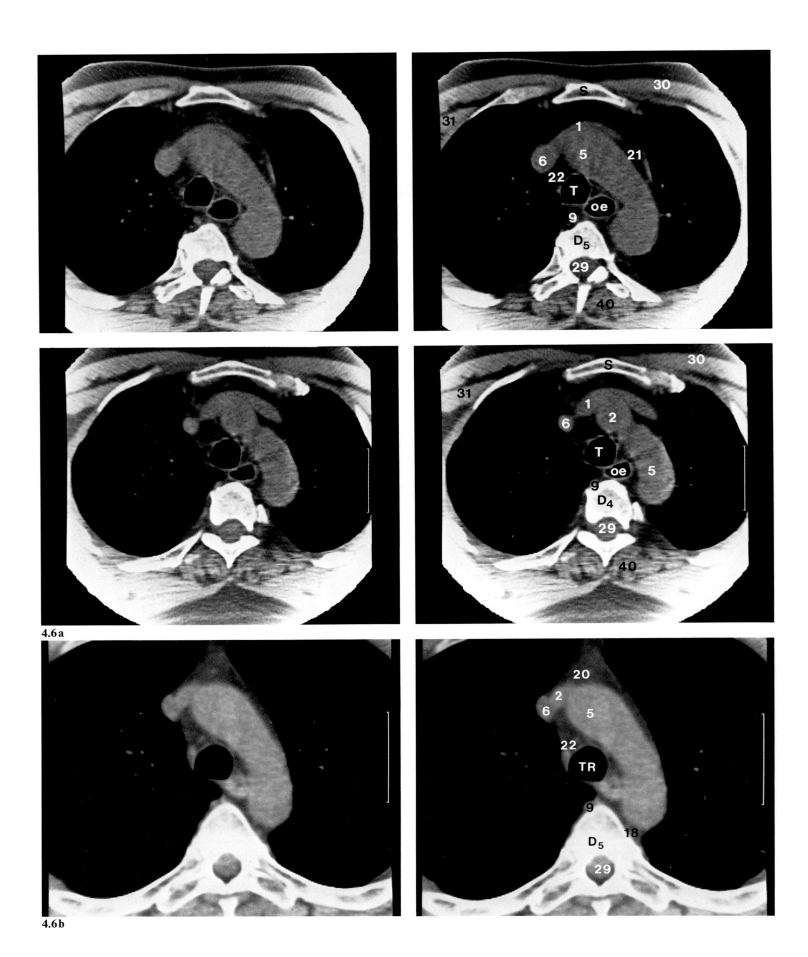

4.6a

4.6b

Fig. 4.6a. Aortic arch level. The scans are first tangential to and then reach the aortic arch; the latter is shaped anteriorly by the brachiocephalic venous trunk, which has a practically horizontal course. This trunk joins its much more vertical right homologue to compose the superior vena cava, which bulges at the external border of the mediastinum, pressing back the pleura. A small vascular structure in front of the spine corresponds to the intercostal vein.

The oesophagus is here distended by air deglutition during the realization of the image. The thinness and regularity of its wall are to be noted. Normal lymph nodes of the left, anterior, mediastinal group, again small, are poorly characterized. They appear as small hazy opacities in the fatty space anterior and lateral to the aortic arch. On the right, the posterior pulmonary penetrates behind the trachea until covering the border of the oesophagus (this disposition explains the formation of the para-oesophageal line in standard radiography). In front of the brachiocephalic venous trunk, the fatty area corresponds to the thymic space. The Barety space which contains the right laterotracheal chain lymph nodes, is to be found behind the vena cava, between the mediastinal pleura, the aorta and the trachea

1	Brachiocephalic vein
5	Aorta
6	Superior vena cava
9	Right superior intercostal vein
21	Left anterior mediastinal lymph node group
22	Right tracheobronchial lymph node group
29	Spinal cord
30	Pectoralis major muscle
31	Pectoralis minor muscle
40	Transversospinalis muscle
T	Trachea
oe	Oesophagus
S	Sternum

Fig. 4.6b. Aortic arch level

2	Brachiocephalic artery
5	Aorta
6	Superior vena cava
9	Right superior intercostal vein
18	Intercostal vein
20	Right anterior mediastinal lymph node group
22	Right tracheobronchial lymph node group
29	Spinal cord
TR	Trachea
oe	Oesophagus

65

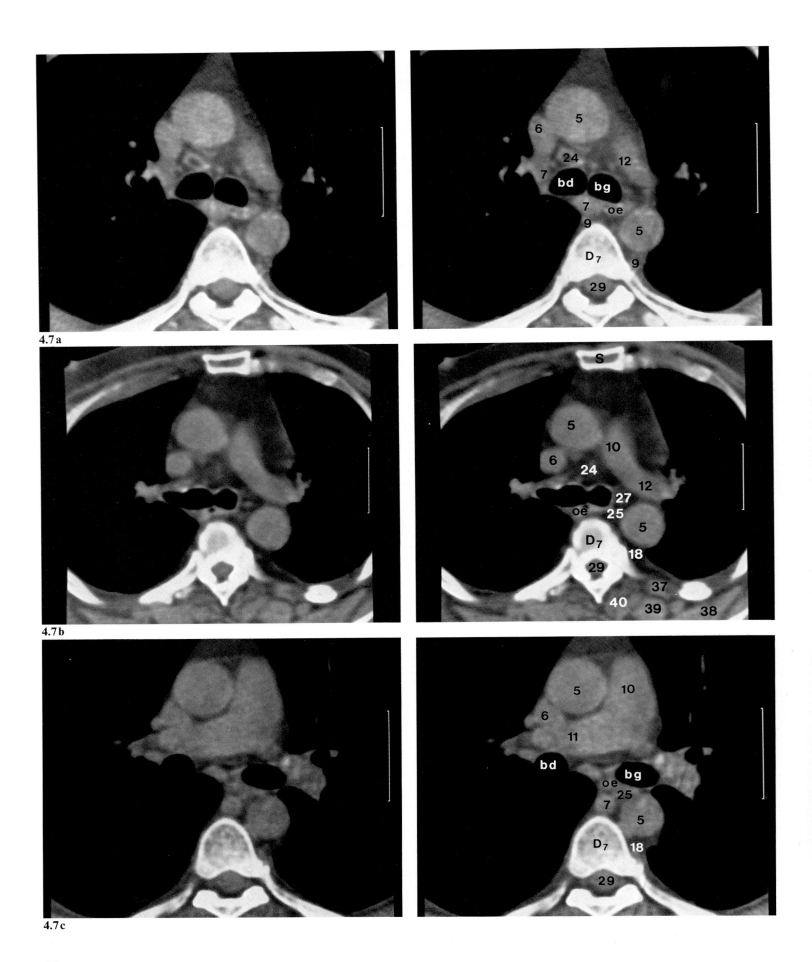

4.7 a

4.7 b

4.7 c

Fig. 4.7a. Tracheal bifurcation level. These images are realized at the height of T 7. The carina tracheae is quite visible, as is the angulation difference of the two primary bronchi, the right one being cut at a higher level than the left, which is more vertical. Anteriorly, the aorta, the superior vena cava and the left pulmonary artery are well individualized. To the front of the bronchial bifurcation, in a fatty space, are situated local lymph nodes which are clearly apparent because of their quite considerable size. Anteriorly it is possible to see, at various heights, fusion of the pleural membranes, the lungs converging to such an extent that they are practically in contact. Great individual anatomical variation is encountered here in accordance with the amount of adipose tissue and the general structure of the thorax. The azygos vein encircles the oesophagus in descending, thus coming around to its posterior face. Here also, the normal oesophageal borders with anterior structures (bronchi) are ill-defined. On the other hand, its borders with the posterior osseous plane and the azygos vein are well identified.

Lower (Fig. 1 b), the pulmonary artery and its posterior "y" bifurcation can be seen

5 Aorta
6 Superior vena cava
7 Azygos vein
9 Right superior intercostal vein
12 Left pulmonary
24 Intertracheobronchial lymph node group
29 Spinal cord
bd Right primary bronchus
bg Left primary bronchus

Fig. 4.7b. Tracheal bifurcation level

5 Aorta
6 Superior vena cava
10 Pulmonary artery
12 Left pulmonary artery
18 Intercostal vein
24 Intertracheobronchial lymph nodes
25 Thoracic duct
27 Bronchopulmonary lymph node
29 Spinal cord
37 Intercostal muscle
38 Rhomboid major muscle
39 Longissimus thoracis muscle
40 Transversospinalis muscle
bi Tracheal bifurcation
S Sternum

Fig. 4.7c. Tracheal bifurcation level

5 Aorta
6 Superior vena cava
7 Azygos vein
10 Pulmonary artery
11 Right pulmonary artery
18 Intercostal vein
25 Thoracic duct
29 Spinal cord
bd Right primary bronchus
bg Left primary bronchus

67

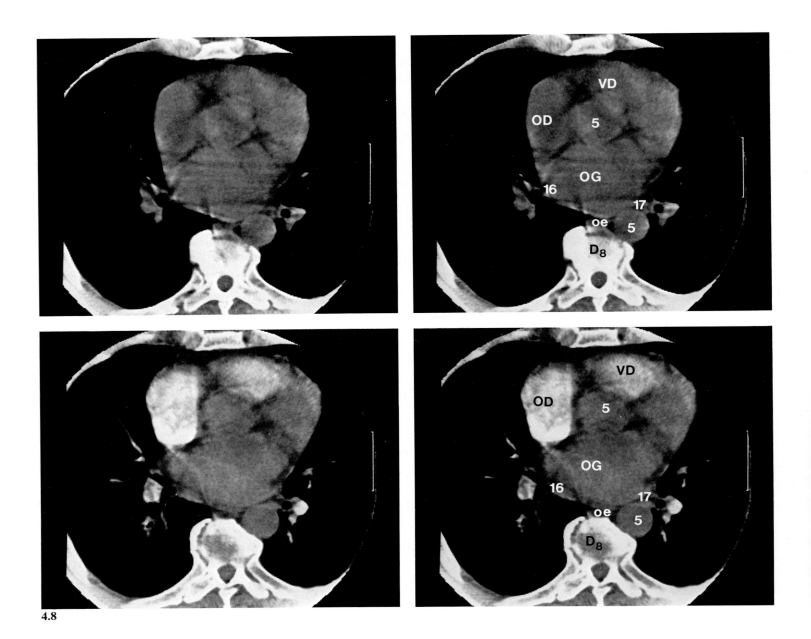

4.8

Fig. 4.8. Left atrial level. These images, realized in rapid sequence at the height of T 8 after i.v. injection of 50 cc contrast medium, illustrate the superior cardiac level. Anteriorly, the upper portions of the right atrium and right ventricle are quite distinguishable from the ascending aorta, being separated from it by mediastinal pleural reflection and fatty tissue. Posteriorly, the left atrium appears as a large oval opacity lying transversely. The close contact between the oesophagus and (a) the left atrium (anteriorly) and (b) the azygos v. (posteriorly) can be seen. The pericardium is generally not visual- ized, whereas the entrance of the pulmonary vein into the left atrium is usually quite visible

5	Aorta
16	Right superior pulmonary vein
17	Left inferior pulmonary vein
oe	Oesophagus
OD	Right atrium
VD	Right ventricle
OG	Left atrium

68

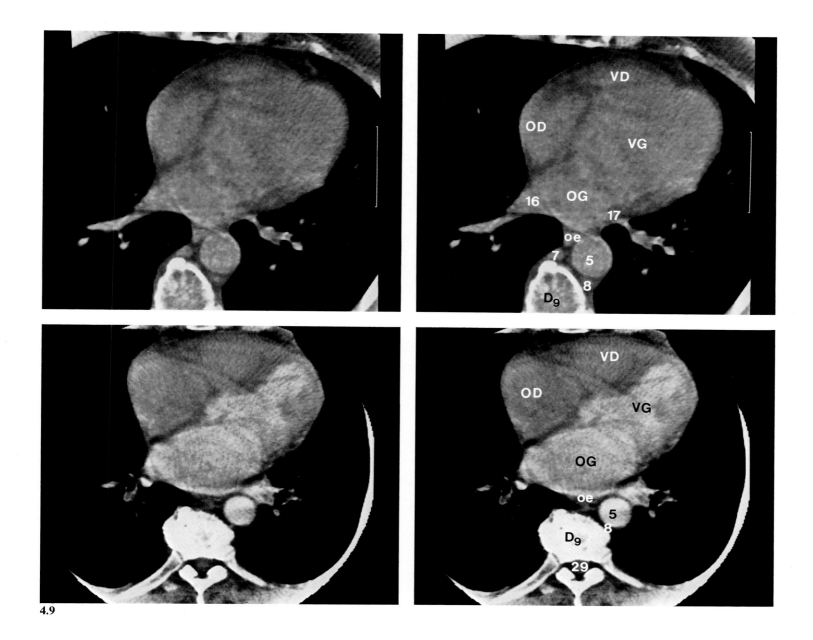

Fig. 4.9. Left ventricular level. Images realized at the height of T 9 after rapid i.v. injection of contrast medium.

The left cavities are opacified. Representation of the heart itself is impaired by the frequency of the heartbeat and by the weak densitometric differentiation of the blood from the cardiac muscle; consequently it is generally difficult to estimate the limits of the cavities and the wall thickness without the aid of contrast medium. In favourable cases, nevertheless, the interventricular and interauricular septa are recognizable. These septa are fairly continuous, being obliquely orientated from front to back and left to right

5	Aorta
7	Azygos vein
8	Hemiazygos vein
16	Right superior pulmonary vein
17	Left inferior pulmonary vein
29	Spinal cord
oe	Oesophagus
OD	Right atrium
VD	Right ventricle
OG	Left atrium
VG	Left ventricle

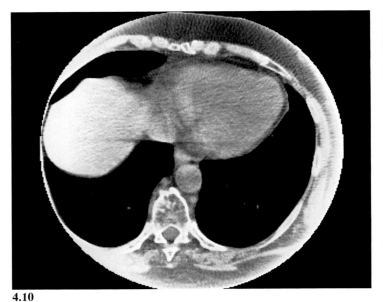 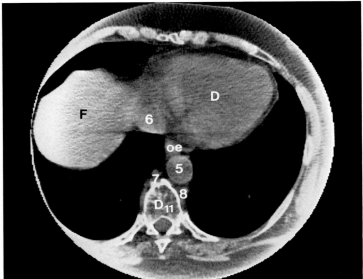

4.10

Fig. 4.10. Inferoposterior mediastinal level. Images realized at the height of T 11. Depending upon the morphological structure of the thorax, the phase of breathing and the axis of the heart, the ventricular opacity gradually blends with the diaphragm caudally if no contrast medium is used

5 Aorta
6 Inferior vena cava
7 Azygos vein
8 Hemiazygos vein

F Liver
D Diaphragm

4.2 Mediastinal Tumours

M. OSTEAUX, A. GRIVEGNEE, T. DARRAS, M. NIJSSENS, P. DE SOMER, P. BIONDETTI, and A.L. BAERT

Computer tomography represents a major advance on conventional radiology in terms of the diagnosis, ascertainment of locoregional extension and follow-up study of mediastinal tumours. The mediastinum, surrounded by its pleural reflections, can be compared to a box—standard plain X-ray films and conventional tomography show the part of the mediastinal tumour projecting beyond the limits of the box, but do not show the inside of the box itself. Oesophageal opacification, arteriography and phlebography are only indirect, poorly sensitive approaches to mediastinal tumours. The superiority of CT in its direct and sensitive demonstration of mediastinal tumours and of their locoregional extension is based on the following technical advantages:

1. *Good densitometric sensitivity,* which allows one to distinguish the tumour from the normal mediastinal structures.
2. *An axial approach,* which allows a favourable topographic representation of lesions so located that conventional radiology would encounter difficulties.
3. *Visualization of the entire topography of an area* in one examination, this being especially useful for the study of tumoral extension.
4. *The possibility of quantitative densitometry,* which enables one to characterize the fatty, calcic, liquid and

cellular components and thus improves diagnosis, permitting a definite diagnosis in some favourable cases (e.g. lipomas).

5. *The possibility of study after i.v. injection of contrast medium,* which permits demonstration of blood vessels, lesion-vascular relationships and vascularization of the lesion itself.

Indications for the use of CT in the mediastinum can be summarized as follows:

1. As a complementary investigation to standard radiography when the latter yields a suspicious or pathological picture; CT is used to establish the presence of the lesion, to obtain morphological or densitometric signs making possible characterization of the lesion and to study locoregional extension.
2. To search for a primary mediastinal lesion suggested by clinical examination despite normal radiological findings (e.g. when a thymoma is suspected in a case of myasthenia).
3. To search for adenopathies in the staging of malignant haemopathies or of some solid tumours (a major indication: CT is very effective in this respect).
4. To search and for locoregional extension for adenopathies in the staging of pulmonary and oesophageal neoplasms.

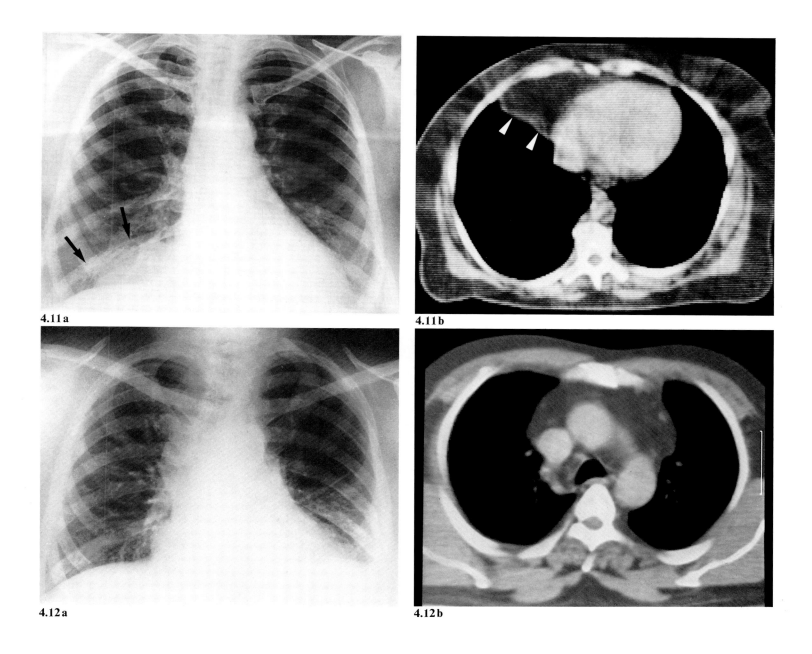

4.11a

4.11b

4.12a

4.12b

Fig. 4.11 a, b. Right pericardial fat pad [52, 54]. **a** PA chest radiograph. **b** Postcontrast scan at heart level. **b** The chest radiograph shows the cardiophrenic angle to be obscured by a prominent shadow (*arrows*). A large mass in the right cardiophrenic angle is seen on the CT scan (*arrowheads*). The cursor reading was −120 HU.

These collections of fat are not usually recognized as radiolucent in the PA roentgenogram. CT can establish the diagnosis by proving the fatty nature of the mass

Fig. 4.12 a, b. Mediastinal lipomatosis [6, 52]. **a** PA chest radiograph. **b** CT scan at level of aortic pulmonary window.

The radiograph and tomogram show widening of the superior mediastinum. CT clearly shows the aortic arch outlined by an accumulation of fat in the anterior mediastinum

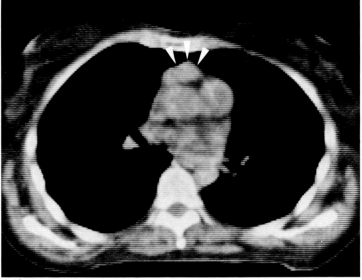

4.13

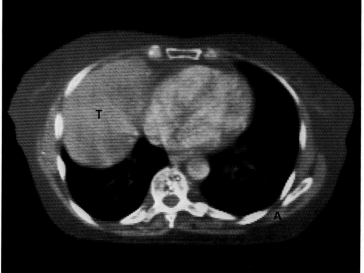

4.14a   **4.14b**

Fig. 4.13. Benign thymoma in a myasthenic patient [2, 53]. This post-contrast tomogram taken at the level of the origin of the great vessels shows a well-defined lobulated mass lying anterior to the aorta and the pulmonary artery, well outlined by surrounding mediastinal fat (*arrowheads*). There is no evidence of invasion of mediastinal structures. This mass was not visualized by conventional radiography.

The discovery of an anterior mediastinal mass in a patient with myasthenia gravis makes surgery mandatory

Fig. 4.14a, b. Thymoma. A contrast-enhanced scan at cardiac ventricular level (**a**) reveals a huge mass of solid density (*T*) in the right pulmonary field. CT shows that this mass is in continuation with the anterior part of the mediastinum (**b**). The attenuation coefficients were compatible with a solid mass.

This case illustrates the fact that if thymoma usually arises in the anterior mediastinum, it can also develop in other compartments

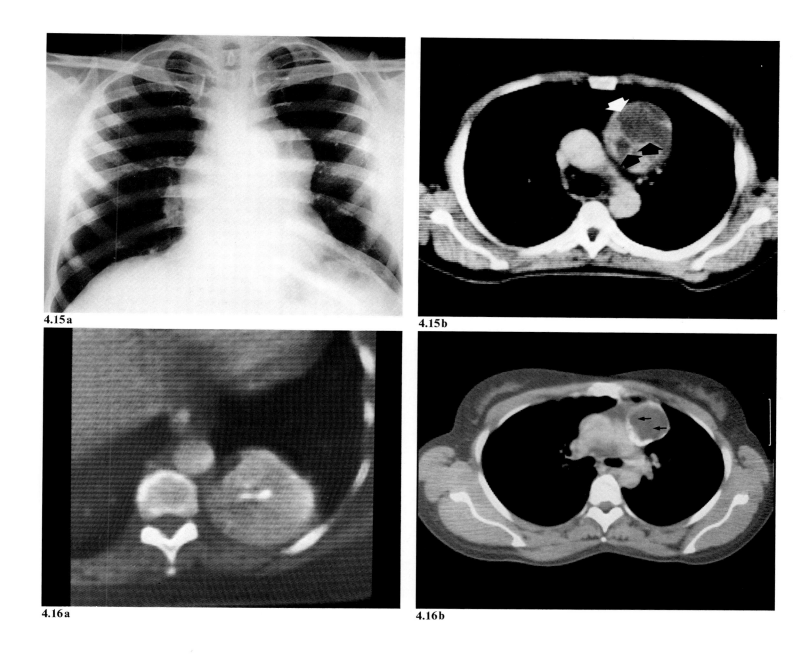

4.15a

4.15b

4.16a

4.16b

Fig. 4.15a, b. Mediastinal teratoma. **a** PA chest radiograph. **b** Post-contrast scan at level of aortic arch.

The radiograph shows a large left mediastinal mass. CT clearly shows a well-delineated, round, inhomogeneous mass containing several areas of decreased attenuation (−10 HU, 0 HU; *arrows*) (fat component). The attenuation values help to establish the nature of the lesion in this case

Fig. 4.16a, b. Teratomas. **a** Contrast-enhanced scan showed a large, round mass of heterogeneous composition. There are calcifications in the middle of solid-liquid attenuation values. This mass was situated in the left vertebral space. **b** Other case. Oval mass with well-defined calcified border, adjacent to the aortic arch, showing heterogeneous internal density with small lipidic areas (*arrows*). In this case the pathologist's first comment was "Normal pancreatic tissue"! The content of the teratoma was essentially digestive tissue (stomach, pancreas, liver, etc.)

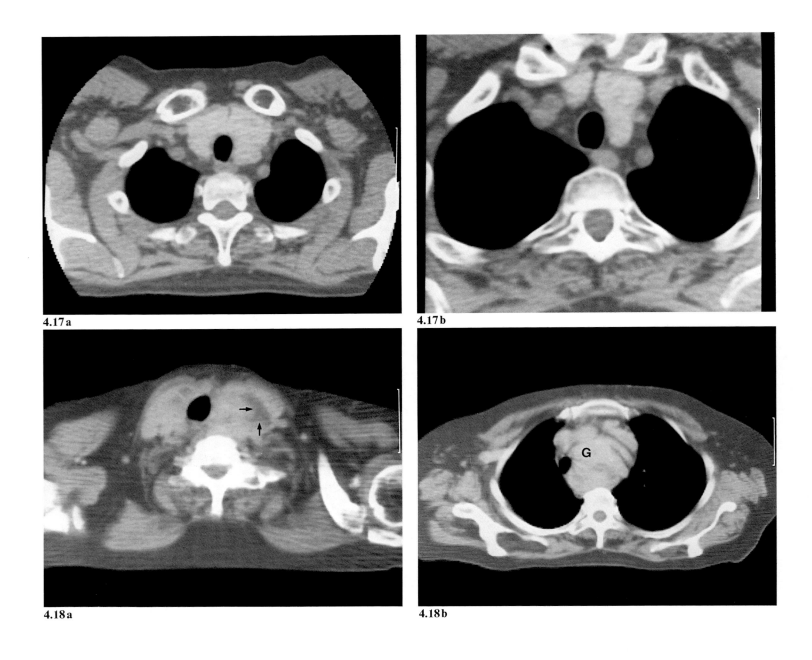

4.17a

4.17b

4.18a

4.18b

Fig. 4.17a, b. Thyroïd hypertrophy (goitre). a Above the manubrium sterni. b At manubrial level. The sections were made at cervicothoracic inlet level without contrast. There is diffuse hypertrophy of the two lobes, more prominent on the left. Note the spontaneous high density of the gland due to the high iodine content

Fig. 4.18a, b. Cervical goitre with endothoracic extension. a Neck level (C7). The heterogeneous mass is located mainly in the left lobe. The hypodense areas represent necrosis (*arrows*). Note the displacement and alteration in shape of the trachea. b The round homogeneous mass (*G*) displaces the trachea, whose diameter is decreased, to the right. Note also the displacement of the anterior vessels

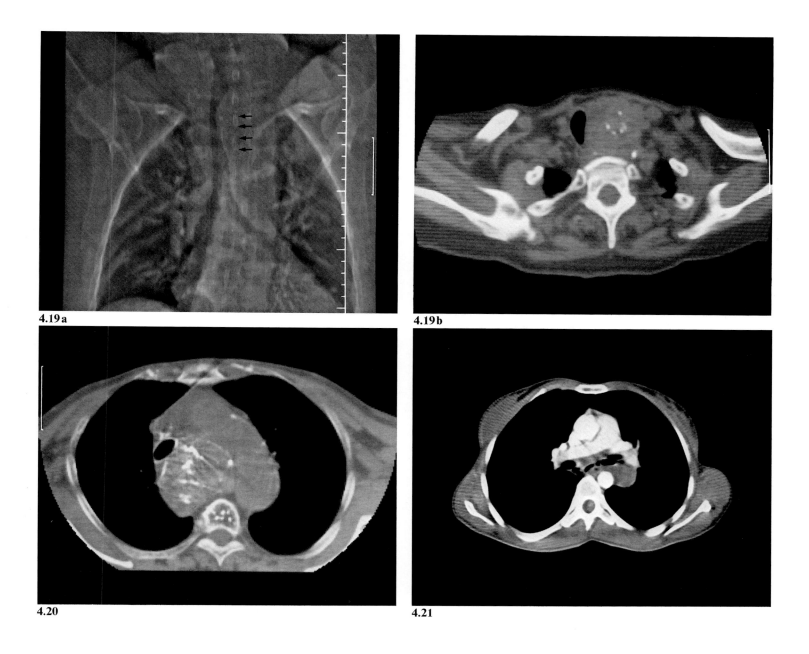

4.19a

4.19b

4.20

4.21

Fig. 4.19a, b. Cervical and mediastinal goitre. a A scout view shows a huge mediastinal mass compressing the trachea, particularly at the level of the cervicothoracic inlet (*arrows*). b At that level, CT shows calcifications in the mass which in this case were not visible on plain films. Note also the good evaluation of tracheal diameter (here markedly reduced)

Fig. 4.20. Calcified endothoracic goitre. Huge and irregular calcifications are shown at aortic arch level (note here again displacement and narrowing of the trachea). This pattern of calcification is highly suggestive of thyroïd goitre

Fig. 4.21. Bronchogenic cyst. This 35-year-old female patient complained of a non-productive cough. CT revealed a mass between the descending aorta descendens and the left pulmonary artery with clear demarcation from these surrounding vascular structures. It has a regular outline and semiliquid attenuation values. There is no clear contrast captation within the lesion after i.v. bolus enhancement, but artefacts make measurement of density unreliable. At thoracotomy the lesion was easily removed, and anatomopathological examination showed it to be a bronchogenic cyst

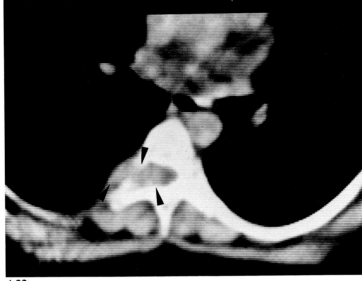
4.22

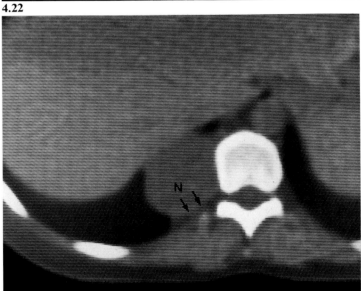
4.23a

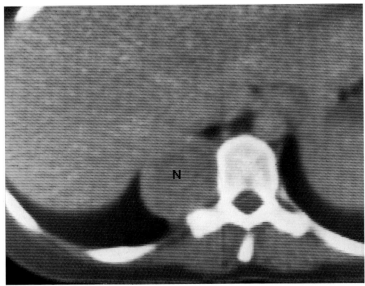
4.23b

Fig. 4.22. Thoracic neurofibroma. This expanded tomogram was taken at the level of T6. The scan demonstrates a fusiform mass (*arrowheads*) posteriorly in the right paraspinal area with destruction of the right pedicle of T6. There is considerable extension of the tumour into the spinal canal.

Enlargement of the intervertebral foramen is clearly demonstrated on the CT image and the intraspinal extension of the lesion may be outlined.

Fig. 4.23a, b. Intercostal schwannoma (neurofibroma). **a** Plain scan. The tumour (*N*) is situated in the right laterovertebral angle. There is no enlargement of the intervertebral foramen. Densitometry reveals solid values. There is a fatty plane between tumour and muscular tissue (*arrows*). **b** Contrast-enhanced scan. There is homogeneous opacification of the mass, revealing no prolongation in the medullary canal. At surgery, there was no cystic degeneration in the mass.

CT is an excellent method for studying lesions in regions difficult to explore with conventional methods (here the laterovertebral region)

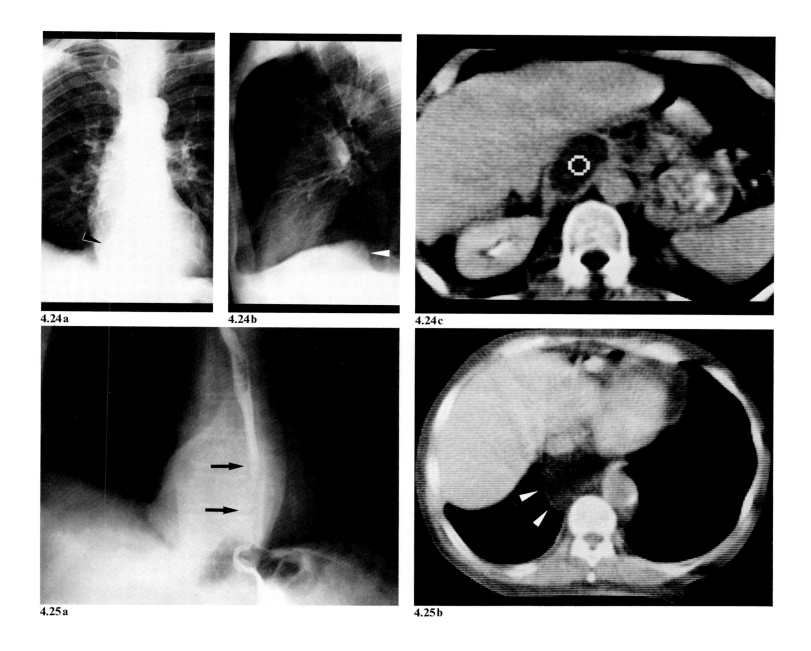

4.24a   4.24b   4.24c

4.25a   4.25b

Fig. 4.24a–c. Right diaphragmatic crural cyst. a PA chest radiograph.
b LL chest radiograph. c Enlarged postcontrast scan at the dome of
the diaphragm. The films show a round retrocardiac mass (*arrows*).
The CT section demonstrates the mass to be a cystic lesion (cursor
reading 10 HU) in the right crus.

A pseudocyst was found in the right crus at intervention

Fig. 4.25a, b. Intrathoracic omental herniation [5]. a PA chest radiograph with oesophageal opacification. b CT scan at the level of the
dome of the right hemidiaphragm. The chest radiograph shows a
retrocardiac mass, displacing the oesophagus to the left (*arrows*). The
CT scan reveals that the retrocardiac mass (*arrowheads*) is composed
of adipose tissue (−120 HU).

The fatty mass represents eventration of abdominal fat through the
diaphragm. In this case CT is diagnostic and can eliminate the need
for other procedures

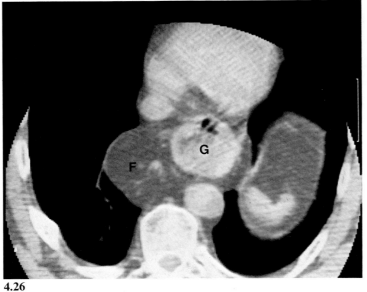

4.26

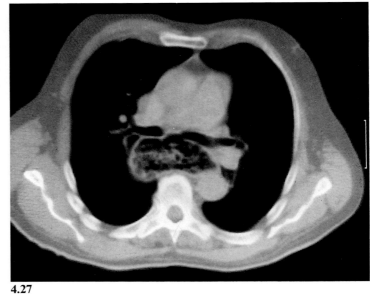

4.27

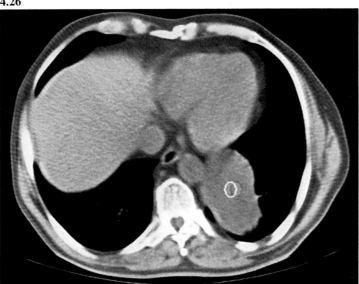

4.28

Fig. 4.26. Hiatus hernia [11, 64]. The scan was taken at the posterior inframinferodiastinal level. There is a huge mass with a regular border and two main densitometric components: a lipidic area representing omental fat (*F*), and a solid, regular, round mass with an air-containing lumen representing the gastric herniation (*G*)

Fig. 4.27. Diverticulum of the oesophagus. The section at supracardiac level revealed a huge mass of the posterior mediastinum, oval in shape with a regular thin wall and a heterogeneous hypodense content.

The diagnosis of oesophageal diverticulum is evident on conventional upper GI tract radiological investigation, but on plain chest films and on tomograms, that condition can sometimes be confused with mediastinal tumour. This patient was referred for staging of a mediastinal tumour

Fig. 4.28. Enterogenic cyst. This mass was found on routine conventional chest radiography in the posterior mediastinum, paravertebrally located on the left. CT shows an oval-shaped lesion with somewhat irregular borders, situated in the posterior mediastinum and connected to the stomach. The mass is homogeneous with sharply demarcated borders and its attenuation values are consistent with fluid. There was no contrast enhancement after intravenous bolus injection of contrast medium.

At thoracotomy a cystic lesion originating from the parietal pleura was easily removed without adherence to aorta or oesophagus. Pathological examination showed a benign enterogenic cyst

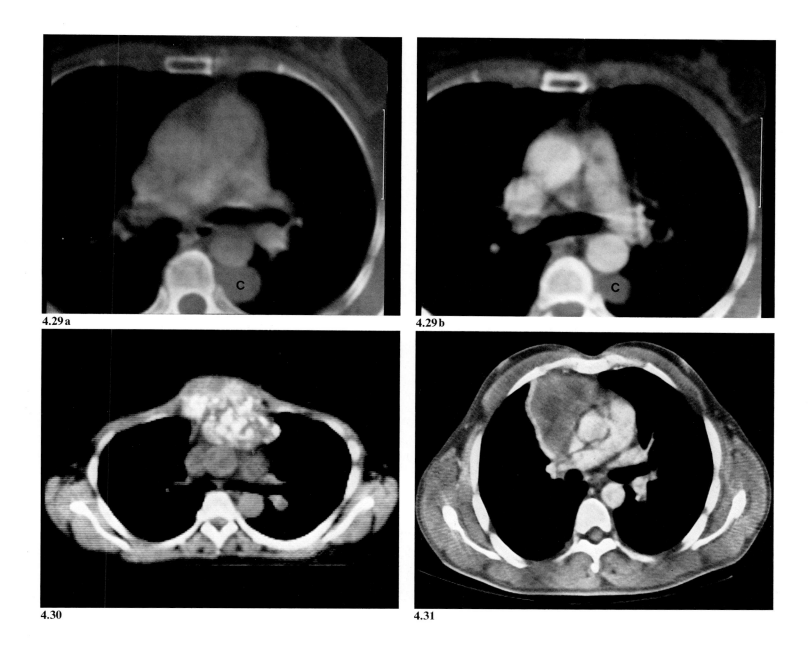

4.29a

4.29b

4.30

4.31

Fig. 4.29a, b. Thoracic duct cyst. **a** A plain scan at the tracheal bifurcation level shows a perfectly round homogeneous mass (*C*) of density 20 HU. **b** A contrast-enhanced scan showed no density enhancement in the mass. Surgery disclosed a thoracic duct cyst, an extremely rare type of posterior mediastinal mass

Fig. 4.30. Sternal osteogenic sarcoma. CT at the level of the carina shows diffuse invasion of the anterior mediastinum by an irregularly calcified mass and posterior displacement of the great vessels.

CT is a reliable method for assessing the intramediastinal extension of the tumour and the presence of pulmonary metastases

Fig. 4.31. Primary seminoma of the mediastinum. This 31-year-old male patient complained of fatigue and shivering.

CT shows an oval-shaped mass with solid attenuation values. The mass is homogeneous and lies very close to the right heart border and ascending aorta, from which structures it cannot be separated. Ventrally, the mass reaches the sternocostal angle. There is slight contrast enhancement after intravenous bolus injection of contrast medium.

Seminoma class V was proven by parasternal percutaneous puncture

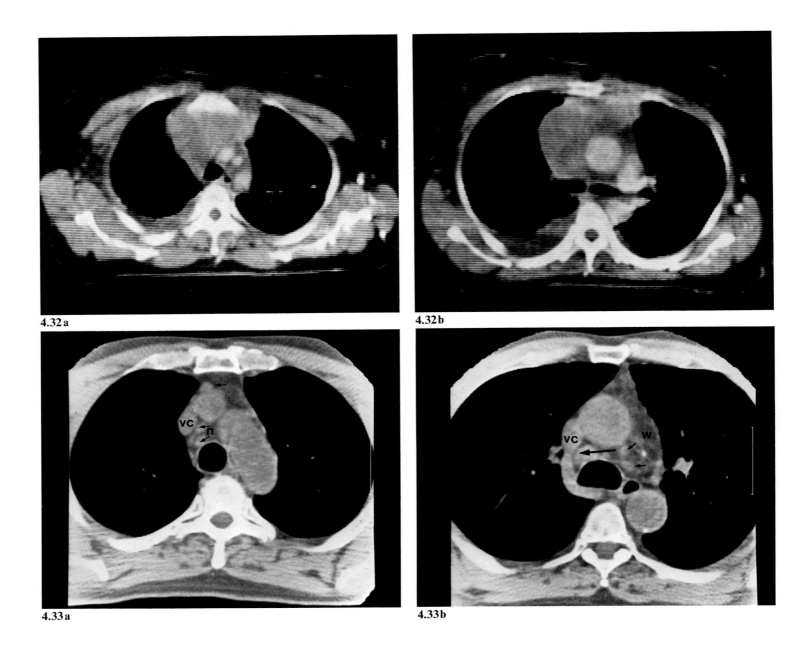

4.32a **4.32b**

4.33a **4.33b**

Fig. 4.32a, b. Malignant epithelioid thymoma [2, 63]. These postcontrast scans are at supra-aortic level (**a**) and at the level of the left pulmonary artery (**b**).

There is extensive tumoral invasion of the mediastinum. The brachiocephalic veins are not recognizable. The superior vena cava is compressed and shows inhomogeneous opacification. The supra-aortic trunks and the trachea are displaced posteriorly. The tumour destroyed the normal fat planes surrounding the aorta and the superior vena cava.

Thoracotomy demonstrated the tumour to be inoperable because of massive invasion of the superior vena cava

Fig. 4.33a, b. Mediastinal polyadenopathies. The sections are at the levels of the aortic arch (**a**) and the azygos arch (**b**). The examination was performed for staging of a non-Hodgkin's lymphoma. There are multiple small adenopathies in the anterior mediastinum in front of the vena cava (*VC*) and the aorta (*arrows*). Also present are adenopathies in the aorto-pulmonary window (*W*) and the pretracheal retrocaval space (*n*). Note the discrete bulge of a bigger node on the azygos arch (*arrow*).

Conventional plain films and tomograms were strictly negative, even a posteriori

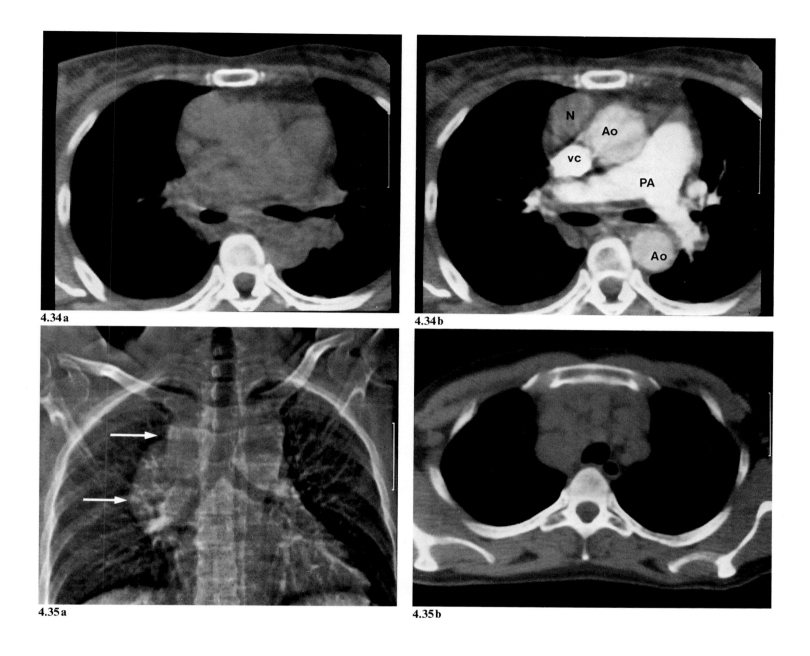

4.34a

4.34b

4.35a

4.35b

Fig. 4.34a, b. Mediastinal Hodgkin's lymphoma. The scans were made at subcarinal level (bifurcation of pulmonary artery). **a** Precontrast. **b** Fifteen seconds after bolus injection of contrast medium. Without contrast, the nodal pathological mass cannot be distinguished from the vascular structures. *N*, node; *Ao,* aorta; *VC,* vena cava; *PA,* pulmonary artery.

This case illustrates the interest of bolus injection of contrast medium in discriminating pathological masses contiguous to vascular structures in the absence of fat interface

Fig. 4.35a, b. Non-Hodgkin's lymphoma: adenopathic masses. Thorax plain film and scout view scan (**a**) display a large mediastinal mass bulging towards the lung at hilar and suprahilar level (*arrows*). CT scan at supramediastinal level (**b**) shows a mass formed by non-confluent nodules of various sizes well delineated by persistent mediastinal fat.

In this case, in the absence of contrast medium it is impossible to distinguish the vessels from mediastinal adenopathies

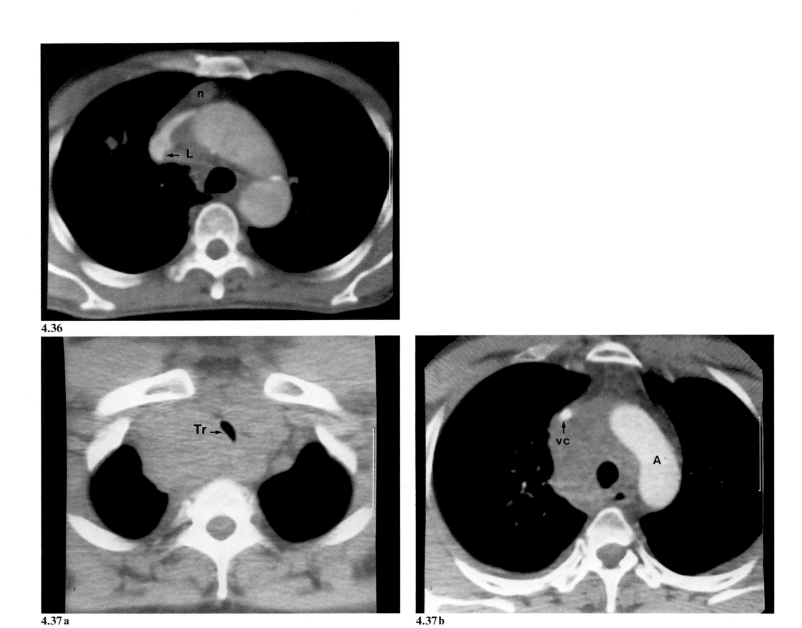

4.36

4.37a

4.37b

Fig. 4.36. Hodgkin's lymphoma with partial occlusion of vena cava. The section was made at the level of the aortic arch during injection of contrast medium into the left brachiocephalic vein. A lymphomatous mass (L) with indistinct borders is responsible for dislocation and partial obstruction of the superior vena cava (←). There is an isolated adenopathy in the anterior mediastinum (n)

Fig. 4.37a, b. Hodgkin's superior mediastinal mass. Sections were made at the levels of the cervicothoracic inlet (a) and the aortic arch with bolus injection of contrast medium (b). In this case the lymphomatous mass is aggressively infiltrating the mediastinal structures. Note the severe narrowing of the trachea (Tr → ; the patient suffered from severe dyspnoea). In b injection of contrast medium reveals repulsion of the aorta (A) and a subtotal stenosis of the vena cava (V.C. →). Lymphomas, namely non Hodgkinian lymphocytic forms, can severely infiltrate adjacent structures. The appearance in this case is very similar to that in lymphoepithelial thymoma

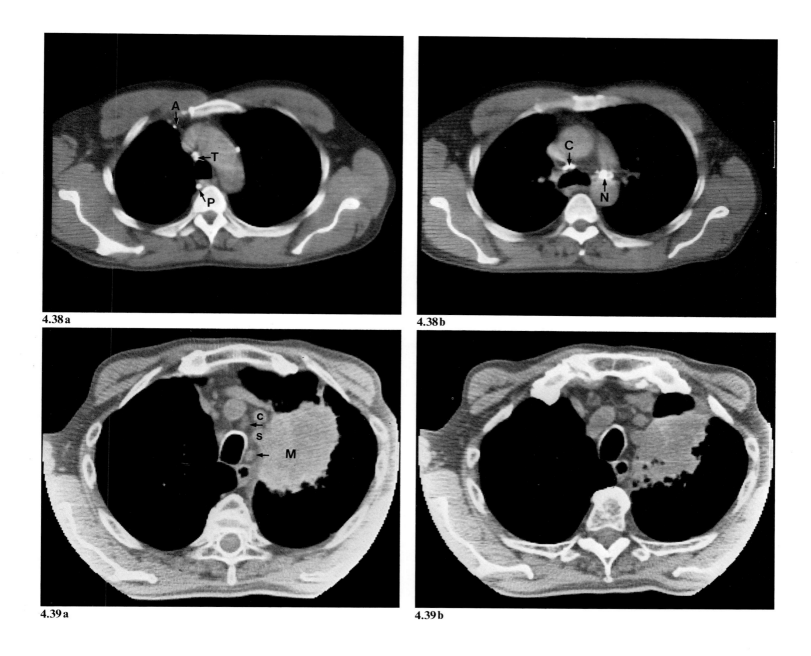

4.38 a

4.38 b

4.39 a

4.39 b

Fig. 4.38a, b. Calcified adenopathies. There are post-tuberculous calcifications of all lymph node groups in the mediastinum (shown here
as a guide to their CT location). a A scan at aortic arch level shows
the anterior mediastinal lymph nodes (A) in front of the great vessels
(here the aorta), the right pretracheal and laterotracheal group in
the retrocaval space (T) and the posterior latero-oesophageal group
(P). b At the level of the aortopulmonary window the precarinal group
(C) and the inferior nodes of the aortopulmonary (left laterotracheal)
group (N) are seen

Fig. 4.39a, b. Invasion of mediastinum by a primitive lung neoplasm.
a A huge neoplastic pulmonary mass (M) is invading the mediastinal
fat and the left subclavian artery (s). The carotid artery (c) is respected. The small "added" opacities (arrows) correspond to adenopathies. b A section 1 cm higher than a shows the absence of adenopathic opacities, making evident their non-vascular nature. (By inte-
grating the images of adjacent slices, it is often possible to discriminate
vascular opacities from adenopathies without bolus injection of contrast medium.)

The clinical value of CT in staging lung carcinoma is still question-
able, due to the relative specificity of CT locoregional invasion cri-
teria. Moreover, visualization of enlarged lymph nodes does not necessarily imply their neoplastic invasion, but can correspond to inflammatory hypertrophy, which is frequently associated with lung neoplasms

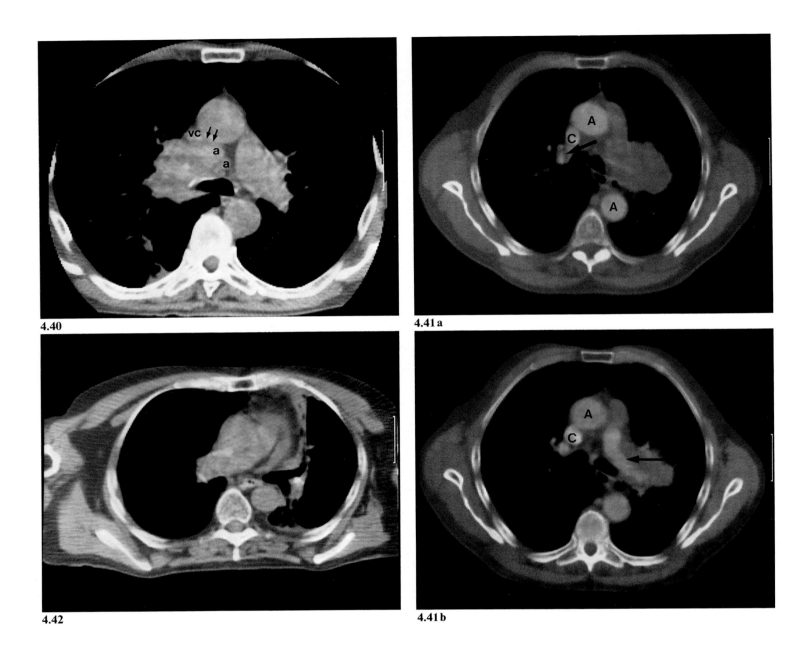

4.40

4.41 a

4.42

4.41 b

Fig. 4.40. Hilar and mediastinal invasion by a lung neoplasm. The section at the level of the carina shows a huge hilar mass infiltrating the mediastinum between the ascending aorta and the bronchial bifurcation. Note the persistence of a fatty interface between tumour and aorta (*arrows*) and the presence of adjacent adenopathies (*a*). *vc*, vena cava.

Hilar neoplasms are often difficult to distinguish radiologically from their adjacent adenopathies

Fig. 4.42. Mediastinal post irradiation fibrosis. The sections are at supracardiac level. The examination was performed 6 months after radiotherapeutic irradiation complementary to surgery for lung carcinoma.

The mediastinum is displaced to the left. The posterior pleural thickening is "in line" with mediastinal condensation. There is left fibrotic condensation with an irregular but globally linear anteroposterior border, which corresponds to the radiotherapeutic field in a pathognomonic feature of post irradiation fibrosis

Fig. 4.41 a, b. Left pulmonary artery invasion by a lung neoplasm. Sections were made at carinal level 15 s (**a**) and 20 s (**b**) after the beginning of injection of contrast medium into the brachiocephalic vein. **a** Opacification of the ascending and descending aorta (*A*), the vena cava (*C*) and the right branches of the pulmonary arteries (*arrow*). There is no opacification of the left branches of the pulmonary arteries. **b** Tardive opacification of the left pulmonary artery (*arrow*), which is included and invaded by the neoplasm

84

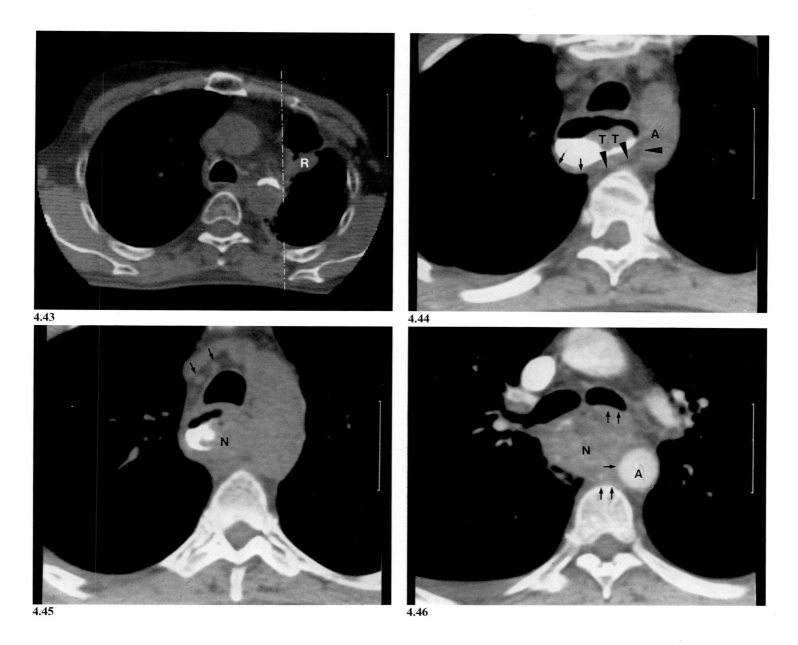

4.43

4.44

4.45

4.46

Fig. 4.43. Post irradiation fibrosis and neoplastic relapse of lung carcinoma. The section is at the level of the azygos arch.

An oval irregularly shaped mass (*R*) extends beyond the external border of the radiotherapeutic field (*broken line*). Note the mediastinal shift to the left, the widening of the anterior fat pad between the pleural reflections, and the global volume decrease of the left hemithorax. There is atheromatous calcification of the descending aorta

Fig. 4.45. Mediastinal invasion by an oesophageal neoplasm. The scan was taken at aortic arch level after the patient had swallowed diluted Gastrografin (meglumine diatrizoate).
There is a large oesophageal mass (*N*) with an irregular lumen. Note the absence of fat interface between the tumour and the trachea anteriorly, the aortic arch laterally. Note also the presence of small adenopathies (*arrows*) posterior to the right brachiocephalic vein.

The absence of a fat interface does not necessarily imply locoregional invasion: a thin fat interface can be missed because of the average effect. Therefore it is important to use thin slices in this application. (In this case locoregional extension was proved at surgery)

Fig. 4.44. Non-invasive neoplasm of the oesophagus. The section was made at the superior mediastinal level, after the patient had swallowed diluted Gastrografin (meglumine diatrizoate). The scan shows global dilatation of the oesophagus with endoluminal tumoral proliferation (*T*), and thickening of the posterior and posterolateral oesophageal walls (*arrows*). Note the persistence of a fatty interface (*arrowheads*) between oesophagus and vertebral structures, and, to the *left,* the aorta (*A*)

Fig. 4.46. Aortic infiltration from oesophageal carcinoma. The section was made at the carinal level 15 s after bolus injection of contrast medium into the brachial vein. A huge posterior mediastinal mass (*N*) is clearly invading the prevertebral plane posteriorly, the bronchial bifurcation anteriorly and the descending aorta (*A*) laterally (*arrows*).
Note the deformation, small reduction of calibre and ill-defined border of the opacified descending aorta

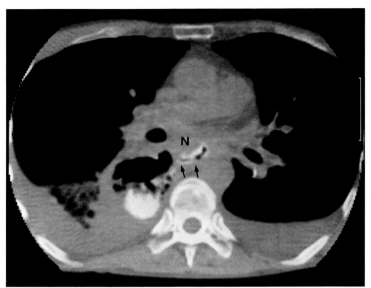

4.47

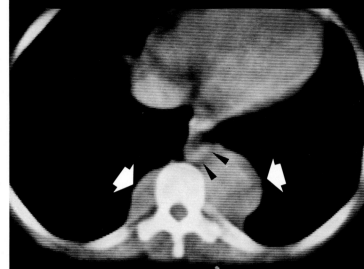

4.48

Fig. 4.47. Mediastinal, pleural and pulmonary extension of oesophageal neoplasm with fistula. The scan was taken at supracardiac level (pulmonary artery bifurcation) after the patient had swallowed diluted Gastrografin (meglumine diatrizoate). A huge posterior mediastinal mass (*N*) is evident between the main bronchi and the aorta without fat interfaces. There is a free-fluid pleural effusion to the *left*. The large pulmonary and pleural solid mass to the *right* is in continuity with the mediastinal tumour. The contrast shows a communication (*arrows*) between the oesophageal lumen and an adjacent cavity in the lung (fistula).

In this case, it is impossible to discriminate the true neoplastic extension from inflammatory lesions secondary to the fistula

Fig. 4.48. Extramedullary haematopoiesis in a thalassaemic patient. The expanded postcontrast scan at heart level shows two masses in the paraspinal area along the lower thoracic spine (*arrows*). There is no evidence of invasion of periaortic fat (*arrowheads*). The density of the mass is 110 HU.

Extramedullary haematopoiesis is associated in most cases with some form of chronic haemolytic anaemia. The masses are highly vascular and present high density after contrast enhancement. The diagnosis should be established by open biopsy, as the masses tend to bleed profusely when incised

4.3 Mediastinal Vascular Pathology

H. Hauser

4.3.1 Introduction

There is a close relationship between the CT exploration of mediastinal vascular structures and the progress in CT technology (discussed in earlier chapters).

Not only has CT scanning time improved, but the administration of iodine contrast solution has changed. The slow perfusion technique has been dropped in favour of rapid i.v. bolus injections, which may be combined with booster bolus injections or rapid drop perfusions. By these means, reasonable imaging of large vascular structures of the mediastinum and the heart has become possible with CT.

Attempts have been made since 1976 to devise an ECG-gated reconstruction device for CT, in order to reduce cardiac motion artefacts. In vivo studies have yielded cardiac imaging in the end-systolic and end-diastolic phases of the ventricles in normal and pathological conditions, with the principal aim of studying more precisely the myocardium; its density, width, contractability and ischaemic disease.

The angio-CT mode allows a rapid sequence of six to seven images per minute. By additional splitting of each image into three partial images, up to 21 density measurements per minute may be obtained. In this way densitometric curves of the infusion of larger blood vessels or the contrast enhancement of tissues may be established. The future will see further reduction in exposure time to substantially below 1 s, using multiple X-ray tubes, as shown in experiments with the dynamic spatial reconstructor or employing new modalities such as nuclear magnetic resonance.

4.3.2 Technique

All scans from the Geneva University Hospital (scans from other institutions are designated accordingly) have been executed with a Somatom machine (Siemens AG). This is a pure fan beam rotary scanner with 256 movable solid-state detectors. A 256 × 256 matrix is used and represented in 64 grey scale levels; the slice thickness is in general 8 mm, but can be set at 4 mm. With a scan time of 4.5 s, a fast series of four exposures per minute is obtainable. Settings of 120 kV and 230 mAs are used, with a spatial resolution of about 2 mm. The only item of special CT equipment used is an independent evaluation unit (Evaluscope).

Patients must be given clear instructions on the necessity of controlled respiration. In repeated deep inspiration several consecutive images are performed. The depth of each inspiration varies little, which helps to obtain reliably comparable cross sections at the same level.

In the majority of cases, the study is performed in two parts. The first consists of a plain series of adjacent or somewhat spaced cross sections covering the whole area of the suggested pathological process. These images allow a rough delimitation of the size and location of the larger mediastinal structures. Calcifications may be easily detected by their elevated densities and the frequently resulting streak artefacts. The attenuation values of pathological tissues can be established as a basic reference for the postenhancement values. Finally, these images serve to determine the level of the most representative cross section, which will be selected for the first scan after i.v. injection of contrast medium.

Crucial in obtaining maximum information are the precise timing of the i.v. contrast injection (in the form of a rapid bolus) and the subsequent exposure of the first postcontrast image, according to the presumed circulation time. The rapid bolus injection of 60 ml of a 76% iodine solution (e.g. meglumine) is executed via a 16-gauge needle into a cubital vein within 3 s. If the right heart cavities or the pulmonary arteries are to be optimally opacified, the first exposure has to be started immediately after injection (Fig. 4.89a); a second scan 20 s after injection of the bolus will selectively opacify the left cavities and the thoracic aorta (Figs. 4.62b, 4.63, 4.89b).

If the left cardiac chambers or the ascending aorta are the site of the pathological process, the first scan should be begun 12 s after the end of the bolus injection (Fig. 4.49).

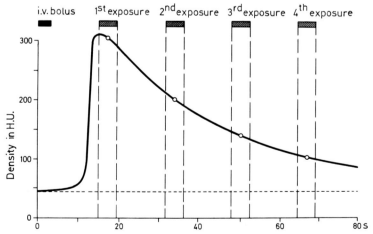

Fig. 4.49. Density distribution during the passage of an i.v. bolus of contrast medium (60 ml in 3 s). The absorption-values expressed in H.U. are measured in the ascending aorta during four exposures at a rate of 4 per minute

87

In case of cardiac malformations with shunt, a very early first scan may indicate the direction and importance of the shunt (Figs. 4.59, 4.60). With abnormal, delayed circulation time it will be the second, third or even fourth image which will demonstrate the passage of the bolus through the cardiac cavities. It is then easy to follow any additional injection by the properly calculated delay before the first exposure. Methods for precise timing, described in the literature, use the heart rate of the patient to calculate the exposure delay according to the area to be studied [70].

If the pathological processes extend over a large area, multiple i.v. bolus injections may be performed. Alternatively, the first i.v. bolus may be followed by a rapid drop infusion of iodine solution (100 ml) in order to maintain a relatively constant, elevated opacification of the vascular structures (e.g. 120–140 HU for 5–7 min) after the initial bolus peak.

The latter technique is preferable in any complete exploration of the cardiac cavities, e.g. while searching for an intracardiac thrombosis. Manipulation, magnification and subtraction of data, coronal or sagittal reconstructions and special density or distance measurements may be required in order to establish the final CT diagnosis in a cardiac disorder or a great thoracic vessel disease.

4.3.3 Indications

Cardiac CT should only be performed when less invasive and less expensive methods cannot provide information precise enough for the appropriate treatment to be chosen.

4.3.3.1 Heart

Cardiac Cavities and Valvular Disease

Parietal and valvular calcification
Single- or multiple-chamber dilatation (degree, size, form)
Local dilatation (cardiac aneurysm)
Pressure overload with myocardial hypertrophy via volume overload with chamber dilatation
Local hypertrophy, as in subvalvular aortic stenosis
Septum deviation, septum defect

Myocardium

Hypertrophy via atrophy
Calcification
Infarcted myocardium (site, extension, evolution)
Hypokinetic and akinetic areas (by ECG gating)

Diffuse myocardiopathy, as in glycogen storage disease
Infiltration by adjacent neoplasm

Intracardiac Space-Occupying Lesions

Intracardiac thrombi associated with myocardial infarction, cardiac aneurysm, valvular disease, cardiac insufficiency
Myxoma
Intracardiac primary neoplasm or metastasis
Cardiac echinococcus

Coronary Arteries

Calcification
Aneurysm
Aortocoronary bypass patency

Pericardium

Total or partial agenesis
Pericardial cyst
Hypertrophy of the pericardial fatty tissue
Calcification
Pericardial thickening (scar, inflammation, postactinic)
Fluid collection (effusion, empyema)
Fresh haemorrhage (tamponade)
Constrictive pericarditis
Primary neoplasm or tumour infiltration by continuity
CT-guided puncture for biopsy or drainage

4.3.3.2 Great Thoracic Arteries

Aortic aneurysm and dissection
Aortic arch malformation
Aberrant arteries (arteria lusoria)
Pulmonary artery dilatation or aneurysm
Pulmonary embolus in the large trunks

4.3.3.3 Great Thoracic Veins

Malformation of the vena cava and azygos, e.g. the azygos continuation in congenital absence of the IVC
Venous dilatation in cardiac insufficiency and obstruction of various origins
Collateral circulation
Peri-oesophageal varices in portal hypertension
Abnormal drainage of pulmonary veins
Stenosis or obstruction by tumoral compression or invasion or by thrombosis
Thrombophlebitis

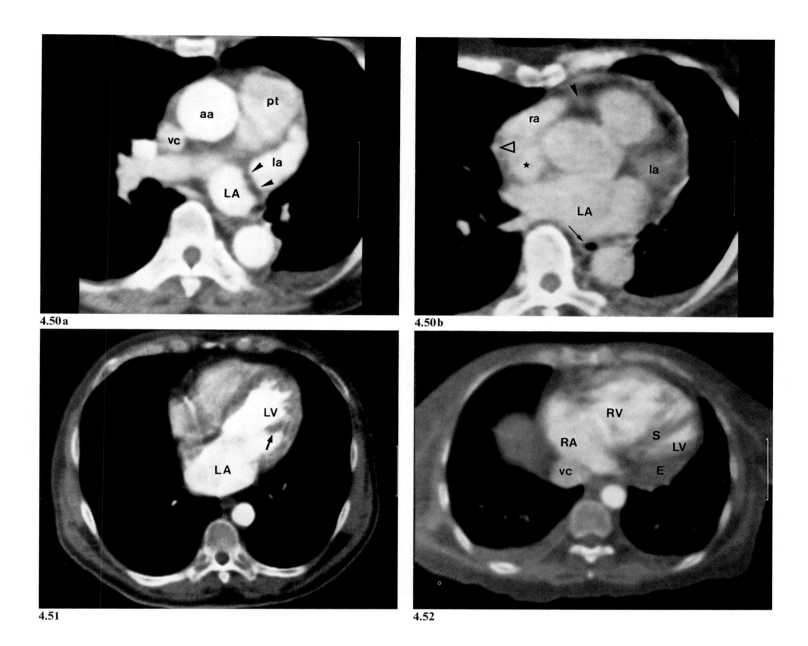

4.50 a

4.50 b

4.51

4.52

Cardiac Cavities and Valvular Disease

Fig. 4.50. a The slightly dilated left auricle (*la*) is separated from the upper pole of the left atrium (*LA*) by a thin fold (►), through which passes the oblique vein of the left atrium. Also shown are the ascending aorta (*aa*), pulmonary trunk (*pt*) and superior vena cava (*vc*). Film taken 15 s after rapid i.v. bolus injection. b The scan shows a slightly dilated right auricle (*ra*) and moderate dilatation of the left atrium (*LA*). At this level the cross section passes through the floor of the left auricle (*la*). The air-filled oesophagus (→) is deviated into the left paravertebral space. The superior vena cava (★) enters the right atrium. Between the right auricle and the pulmonary trunk lies the right coronary artery (►). The small notch (▷) lateral to the right atrium corresponds to the pericardiophrenic vessels, which run close to the phrenic nerve.

Film taken late after i.v. bolus injection

Fig. 4.51. Mitral valve insufficiency. The condition causes a mild dilatation of the left atrium (*LA*), a mild muscular hypertrophy of the left ventricle (*LV*) and, in particular, hypertrophy of the anterior papillary muscle (→).

Films obtained during the passage of the iodine bolus through the left cavities (12 s after rapid bolus injection)

Fig. 4.52. Pulmonary hypertension due to Menocil (aminorex fumarate), associated with insufficiency of the tricuspid valve. There is a significant enlargement of the right ventricle (*RV*), with horizontalization of the interventricular septum (*S*), a small left ventricle (*LV*), a dilated right atrium (*RA*) and inferior vena cava (*VC*) and a small quantity of pericardial effusion (*E*).

The pressure in the right ventricle was elevated to 110 mm Hg during cardiac catheterization and the pressure in the right atrium was measured as 35 mm Hg.

Film obtained after rapid i.v. bolus injection

89

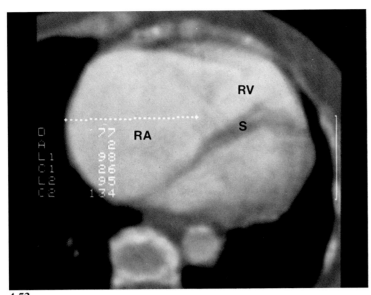

4.53

Fig. 4.53. Tricuspid valve insufficiency. The right atrium (*RA*) is strongly dilated (to 77 mm in transverse diameter). The moderately enlarged right ventricle (*RV*) is displaced to the left and the interventricular septum (*S*) is deviated. Clinically, this patient presented with pulsatile hepatomegaly.

Film taken after i.v. contrast injection

Fig. 4.56a, b. Right heart failure with lower extremity oedema and ▷ stasis of the jugular veins. **a** Combined mitral and tricuspidal insufficiency with marked dilatation of the left and right atria (*LA*, *RA*) is evident. Note also a small aortic valve calcification (→). **b** At this level, the normal ascending aorta (*aa*) and pulmonary trunk (*pt*) are seen in front of the dilated left atrium (*LA*) and the dilated superior vena cava (*vc*)

Film obtained after i.v. contrast injection

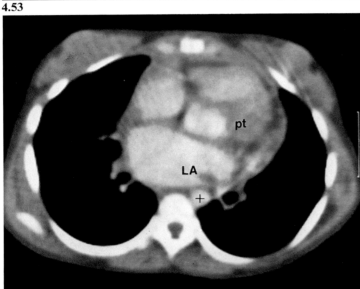

4.54a   **4.54b**

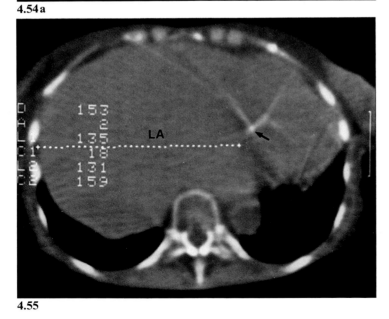

4.55

Fig. 4.54a, b. Mitral valve disease with predominant insufficiency and pulmonary hypertension (same patient as in Fig. 4.94). **a** The left atrium (*LA*) is considerably dilated, the pulmonary trunk (*pt*) enlarged and the descending aorta (+) particularly small (1.2 cm in diameter). **b** The Starr-Edwards prosthesis in the mitral valve position causes streak artefacts.

Film obtained after i.v. bolus injection

Fig. 4.55. Mitral valve insufficiency. The greatly dilated left atrium (*LA*), 15 cm in transverse diameter, occupies the greater part of the thoracic cross section. The vertebral body causes a posterior impression on the left atrium. The mitral valve position is indicated by a single nodular, valvular calcification (→). This study was performed to exclude a paracardial space-occupying lesion such as a cyst or a tumour.

No contrast injection

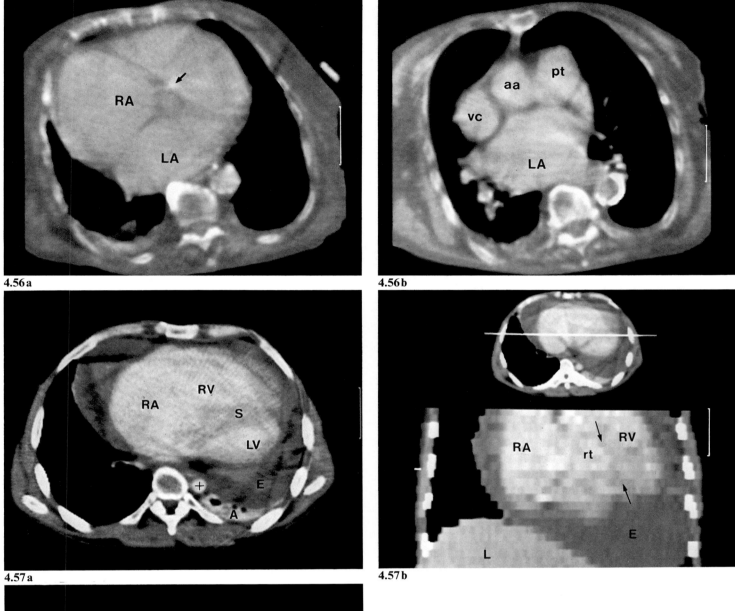

4.56a

4.56b

4.57a

4.57b

4.57c

Fig. 4.57a–c. Ebstein's disease. **a** The markedly enlarged right atrium (*RA*) and right ventricle (*RV*) form the major part of the heart. The small left ventricle (*LV*) is seen posterior to the horizontal septum (*S*). The descending aorta (+) is of small diameter. Note the important pericardial effusion (*E*) and the left posterior lung atelectasis (*A*). **b** In coronal reconstruction display the low insertion of the tricuspid valve is more evident. The right atrioventricular complex is formed by three cavities; the right atrium (*RA*), the atrialized part of the right ventricle (*rv*) and the remainder of the right ventricle (*RV*). The *arrows* indicate the level of the tricuspid valve, which was in this patient 26 cm in circumference. Note the extensive pericardial fluid collection (*E*), located predominantly in the subcardiac region, which is displacing the left lobe of the liver (*L*). **c** The inferior vena cava is dilated to 47 mm in oblique diameter and there is a huge pericardial effusion (2,500 ml).

All films obtained after rapid bolus injection

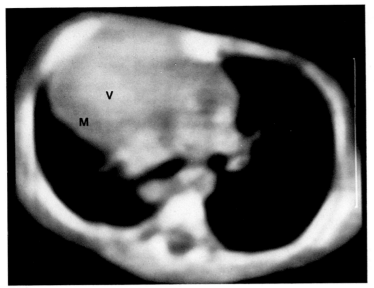

4.58

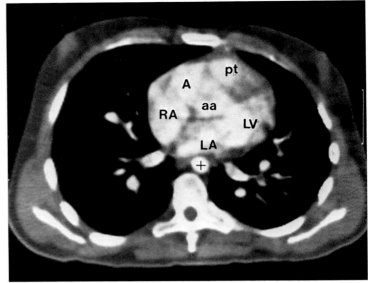

4.59

4.60

Fig. 4.58. Single ventricle and dextrocardia (situs inversus). In this 6-month-old baby the heart is situated on the right. The ventricular mass shows a single cavity (*V*) surrounded by a thickened myocardium (*M*). Note the deformation of the right anterior chest wall. Multiple malformations were associated with mitral valve atresia and atrial septal defect.

Film obtained after i.v. bolus of 8 ml iodine solution, without general anaesthesia

Fig. 4.60. Atrial septal defect with shunt inversion. This film obtained immediately after a rapid bolus injection (3 s) shows a very dense and precocious opacification of the left atrium (*LA*) and the descending aorta (*da*), indicating the importance of the right to left shunt.

Note the prominent anterior wall of the right ventricular outflow path (▶) and the small size of the hilar vessels, the typical signs of pulmonary hypertension, and also the atrial septal defect (→) and the dilated right atrium (*RA*)

Fig. 4.59. Atrial septal defect associated with abnormal drainage of a left pulmonary vein into the right atrium.

Due to the double shunt (predominantly left to right) the film, exposed immediately after rapid i.v. bolus injection, shows inhomogeneous but simultaneous opacification of all cardiac cavities, rather than the consecutive opacification of right and then left cavities which results from normal bolus passage (Fig. 4.89). As a consequence of the shunt there are enlarged pulmonary vessels and a small descending aorta (+).

In addition, this patient had a 4-cm aneurysm (*A*) of Valsalva's sinus, situated anteriorly and to the right of the aortic root (*aa*). The upper part of the right atrium (*RA*) is slightly enlarged; the atrial septal defect itself is not visible at this level. Note also the pulmonary trunk (*pt*), left ventricle (*LV*) and left atrium (*LA*)

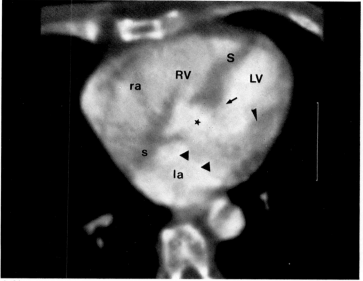

4.61 a

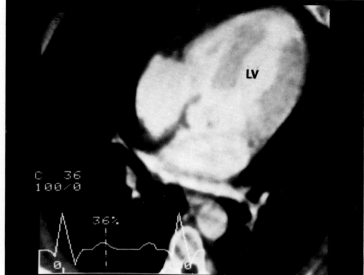

4.61 b

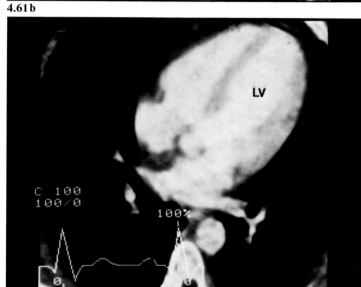

4.61 c

Myocardium

Fig. 4.61 a–c. Normal anatomy. **a** In this cross section at the level of the mitral valve (▲) and the aortic outflow path (★), the myocardium is visualized at the left ventricular wall, the interventricular septum (*S*), the interatrial septum (*s*) and the anterior (►) and posterior (→) papillary muscles of the left ventricle (*LV*). In addition, the right ventricle (*RV*) and the right (*ra*) and left (*la*) atria are visualized. Note the normal oblique position (nearly 45°) of the interventricular septum.

Scan obtained shortly after i.v. bolus injection, during the passage of the dye through the left cardiac cavities.

b End-systolic ECG-gated cardiac cross section. The left ventricular cavity is markedly diminished in its transverse diameter, and the later-al and septal muscular walls are thickened considerably. The left ventricle (*LV*) is contracted, while both atria are filled.

Scan obtained by ECG gating (using the cardio-CT accessory to the Somatom scanner) after i.v. contrast administration (courtesy of Siemens AG, Erlangen).

c End-diastolic ECG-gated cardiac cross section. Both ventricular chambers are filled to their full size and the muscular walls are stretched. Both atria are contracted. *LV*, left ventricle.

Courtesy of Siemens AG, Erlangen

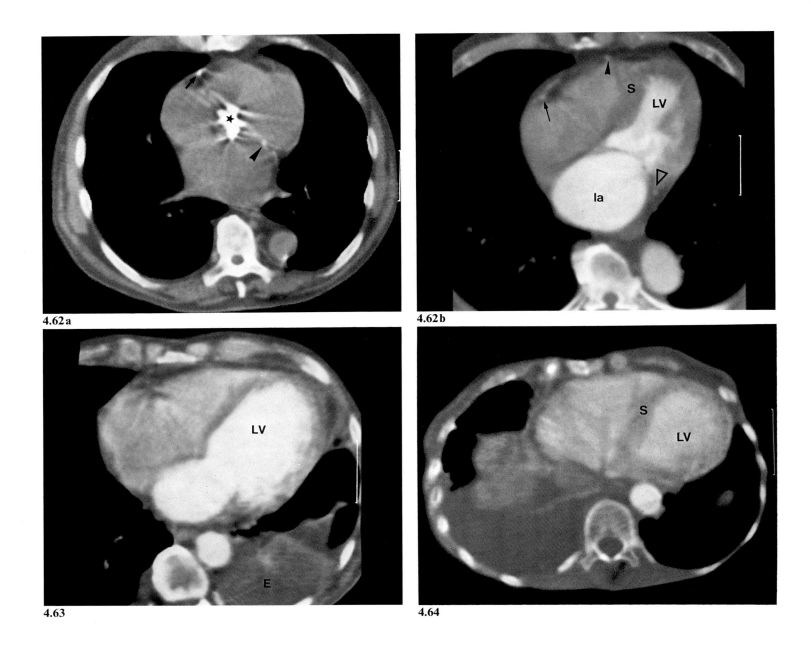

4.62a **4.62b**

4.63 **4.64**

Fig. 4.62a, b. Predominantly stenotic aortic valve disease with associated mitral valve disease. **a** There is extensive aortic valvular calcification (★) and slight mitral valve calcification (➤). The right coronary artery (→) is also calcified, and there is enlargement of the left atrium.

Film obtained without iodine contrast material.

b Considerable hypertrophy of the left ventricular muscle is evident; in fact the transverse diameter of the left ventricular wall and interventricular septum (S) has doubled to 1.6 cm. The interventricular septum is verticalized, the left atrium (la) moderately dilated.
The right coronary artery (→) and the anterior interventricular (➤) and circumflex branches (▷) of the left coronary artery are opacified. The hypertrophied left ventricle (LV) has displaced the anterior interventricular branch towards the midline.

Film taken shortly after a rapid bolus injection with selective opacification of the left cavities

Fig. 4.63. Diffuse ischaemic coronary disease. Atrophy of the myocardium and strong dilatation of the left ventricle (LV) result from the ischaemic condition. Note the left basal pleural effusion (E) due to left heart failure. This patient had a previous infarction in the septal area.

Scan with selective opacification of the left cavities obtained shortly after rapid i.v. bolus injection

Fig. 4.64. Cardiomegaly. There is combined hypertrophy of the myocardium and dilatation of the left ventricle (LV), in a combined aortic and mitral valvular disease. The slightly verticalized interventricular septum (S) is 18 mm in width. Note the prominent left anterior chest wall due to the cardiomegaly, and the right pleural effusion.

Scan obtained after i.v. bolus injection.

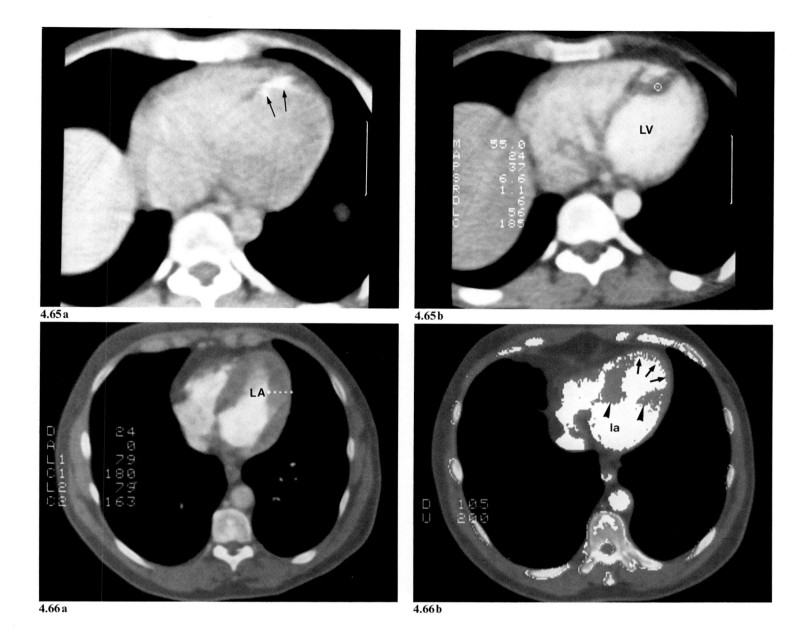

4.65a

4.65b

4.66a

4.66b

Fig. 4.65a, b. Myocardial infarction 10 years prior to this study. No contrast injection. a There is calcification (→) of the myocardium in the anteroseptal part of the left ventricular wall and moderate cardiomegaly. b Same cross section after bolus injection of iodine dye. Adjacent to the myocardial calcification, a thick anteroseptal filling defect (☉) was found in the left ventricle (LV); it was not enhanced by the contrast medium (55 HU), whereas the normal myocardium measured within the septum was enhanced from 50 HU to 90 HU. The lesion is believed to be an organized parietal thrombus on the scar tissue at the site of the infarction. The remainder of the left ventricle is dilated and the ventricular wall is thin due to the diffuse coronary ischaemic disease

Fig. 4.66a, b. Severe coronary disease with two previous infarcts of the anterior wall. a There is hypertrophy of the myocardium of the left ventricle (LV) due to long-standing arterial hypertension. The lateral wall of the upper third of the left ventricle is 24 mm in width. The septum is almost vertical.

Film obtained after rapid bolus injection.

b In the apical region of the left ventricle there is marked local thinning (→) of the anterior wall and local dilatation of the left ventricular cavity, corresponding to an apical cardiac aneurysm. Note the hypertrophied papillary muscles (►) of the mitral valve. la, left atrium.

This scan was obtained after i.v. bolus contrast injection and is displayed in high lighting mode for better demonstration of the apical aneurysm. All densities between 105 HU and 200 HU, shown in *white*, correspond to the opacified blood within the cardiac cavities

95

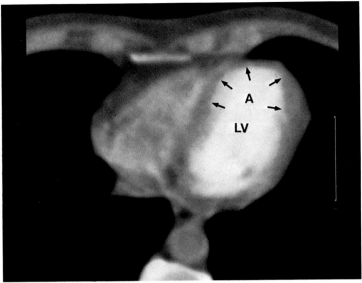

4.67

Fig. 4.67. Previous anteroseptal myocardial infarction complicated by a recidivant Dressler syndrome.

This 55-year-old patient now has an anteroseptal left ventricular aneurysm (*A*). There is a focal widening (→) of the apical part of the left ventricular chamber (*LV*) and concomitant thinning of the anterior muscular wall.

This CT left ventriculogram was obtained 12 s after rapid i.v. bolus injection

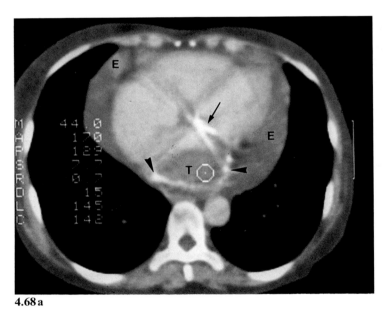

4.68 a

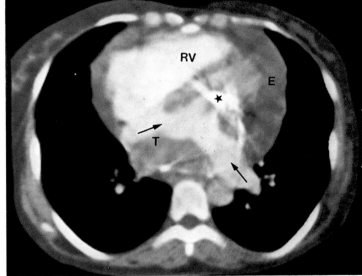

4.68 b

Intracardiac Space-Occupying Lesions

Fig. 4.68 a, b. Subtotal thrombosis of the left atrium in mitral stenosis.
a The large filling defect in the left atrium is not visible on the non-enhanced scan, as its density (37–44 HU) is similar to that of the blood. After i.v. bolus injection, the non-enhancing thrombus (*T*) becomes quite visible.

Note in addition the mitral valve calcification (→), the calcification in the left atrial wall (►) and the concomitant pericardial effusion (*E*).

Scan obtained late after bolus injection.

b Slightly higher cross section. The thrombus (*T*) is situated in the posterior part of the left atrium and represents no obstacle to the flow of blood from the pulmonary veins on either side (→) towards the markedly calcificed mitral valve (★). The thrombosis was an incidental finding in evaluating the pericardial effusion (*E*). *RV*, right ventricle.

Film obtained immediately after i.v. bolus injection

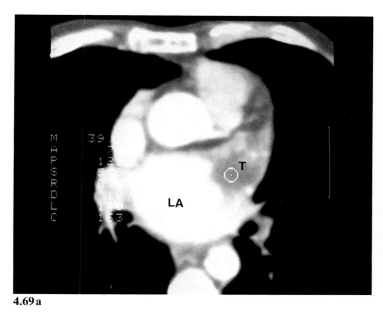

4.69 a

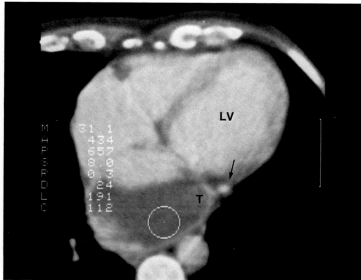

4.69 b

4.69 c

Fig. 4.69 a–c. Mitral disease. **a** There is thrombotic obliteration of the left auricle (*T*) and dilated left atrium (*LA*) due to the mitral disease. The mitral valve had been replaced by a Starr-Edwards prosthesis 3 years previously. The unenhancing thrombus measured 31–39 HU. The patient was under poorly controlled anticoagulation.

Scan obtained shortly after i.v. bolus injection.

b At a lower level, a thrombotic filling defect (*T*; 31 HU) occupies the greater part of the inferior portion of the left atrium. Note a mild dilatation of the left ventricle (*LV*) due to the mitral disease and an opacified venous bypass (→) to the circumflex branch of the left coronary artery. In fact, the patient had a triple aortocoronary

bypass procedure and the atrial thrombosis was an incidental finding during CT control of graft patency. See also Fig. 4.79.

Film obtained late after bolus injection.

c This preoperative control study was undertaken after $2^1/_2$ months well-controlled anticoagulation therapy. There was considerable regression of the left atrial thrombosis and only a small left lateral residual thrombus (*T*) could be visualized. The cardiac operation was cancelled and further CT control of the anticoagulation therapy proposed.

Film obtained after i.v. contrast administration

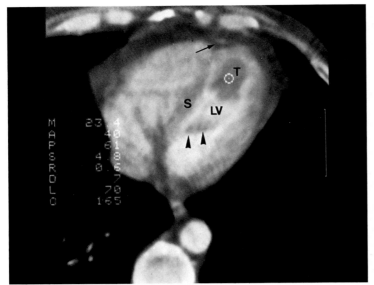

4.70a

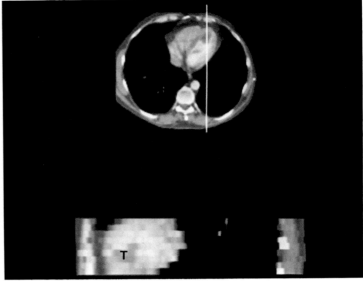

4.70b

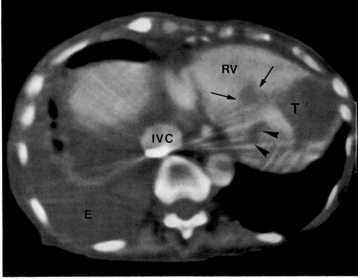

4.71

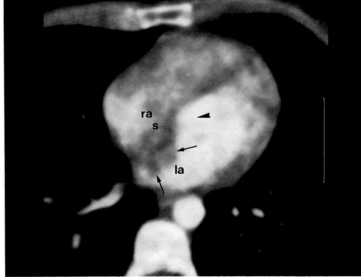

4.72

Fig. 4.70a, b. Previous anterior wall and septal myocardial infarct with recent history of cerebral and peripheral arterial embolic disease.

a This 55-year-old patient had a left ventricular apical thrombus (*T*) attached to the anterior part of the interventricular septum (*S*). The thrombus yielded low densities of 20–30 HU and was 2–3 cm in diameter. Note the posterior cusp of the mitral valve (►) and the anterior

interventricular branch (→) of the left coronary artery. *LV*, left ventricle.
Film obtained during bolus passage through the left cardiac cavities.

b Sagittal reconstruction of the left ventricle from nine adjacent slices, each 8 mm thick. The apical attachment of the intraventricular thrombus (*T*) is visualized

Fig. 4.71. Multiple thrombi within the cardiac ventricles. This 87-year-old lady with dilatation of all cardiac cavities and a history of myocardial infarction 2 years prior to this study was investigated for a significant right-sided pleural effusion (*E*). A huge filling defect (*T*) occupies the apical part of the left ventricle; its low attenuation coefficient of 45 HU is suggestive of a thrombus. A second, smaller thrombus (►) in the left ventricle is attached to the posterior part of the septum. A third lesion (→), also fixed to the septal wall, is situated within the right ventricle (*RV*).

Note the dilated inferior vena cava (*IVC*) containing a depot of contrast solution, which is retained by the slow flow of right heart failure. No arterial embolic disease was observed in this patient.

Film obtained $2^1/_2$ min after i.v. bolus injection

Fig. 4.72. Myxoma in the left atrium. The small, bilobate, hypodense filling defect due to the myxoma (→) has a large base attached to the interatrial septum (*S*). The tumour was 2.5 cm by 1 cm in size (verified at operation) and its insertion into the septum was adjacent to the foramen ovale. This cross section is taken at the level of the aortic outflow path (►). The right (*ra*) and left (*la*) atria are of normal size. Unfortunately the small tumour size and the motion artefacts do not allow exact density measurements.

Scan obtained during the passage of the rapid i.v. bolus of contrast material through the left cardiac cavities

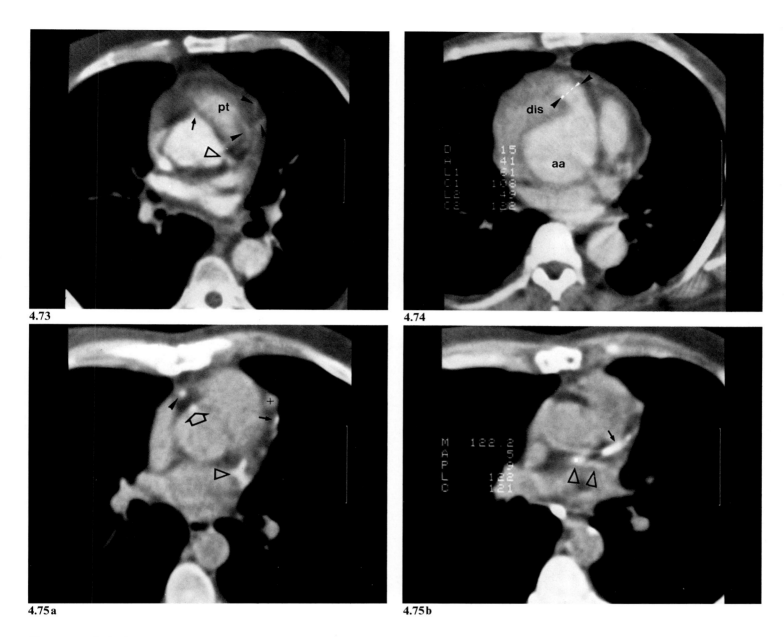

4.73

4.74

4.75a

4.75b

Coronary Arteries

Fig. 4.73 Normal anatomy: the sinuses of Valsalva with the origin of the left coronary artery and the anterior interventricular branches. The supravalvular part of the ascending aorta is of cloverleaf form due to the three sinuses of Valsalva. The main trunk of the left coronary artery (▷) has its origin in the middle of the left sinus.

The three branches (►) of the left anterior interventricular artery are seen to the left of the main pulmonary trunk (*pt*). The origin of the right coronary artery is faintly visible (→) as it branches off the anterior sinus of Valsalva.

Scan taken after i.v. bolus injection

Fig. 4.74. Aneurysm of the right coronary artery at its origin. The transverse diameter of the aneurysm (►) is 15 mm. In addition a dissecting aortic aneurysm (*dis*) is present, surrounding the right coronary artery aneurysm and also the anterior and right lateral part of the ascending aorta (*aa*). This patient has Marfan's syndrome (see also Fig. 4.93).

Scan taken after i.v. bolus injection

Fig. 4.75a, b. Severe three-vessel coronary disease. **a** There is calcification of the right coronary artery (►), the left anterior interventricular branch (→), the circumflex artery (▷) and the aortic wall (⇒). Also visible is a 3-year-old venous bypass (+) to the anterior interventricular branch, which the study proved to be occluded.

Scan taken without i.v. contrast injection.

b At a slightly higher level, a thick, long calcified plaque is present in the proximal part of the anterior interventricular artery (→). Note a transverse linear structure posterior to the ascending aorta; this is a venous graft to the circumflex artery (▷) situated in the transverse pericardial sinus. The density of the bypass was 122 new HU, signifying arteriosclerotic calcification of the arterialized venous wall.

Film obtained without i.v. contrast. The graft appeared to be patent after i.v. bolus injection

99

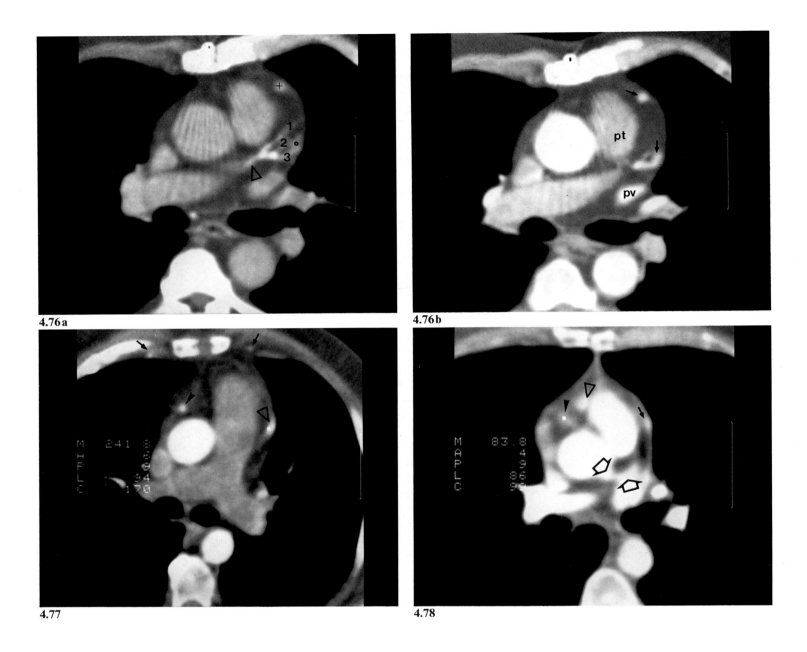

4.76a

4.76b

4.77

4.78

Fig. 4.76a, b. Two-vessel coronary disease. a Dense calcifications are present at the bifurcation of the left main coronary trunk (▷) into the anterior interventricular (1) and circumflex (3) arteries, as well as at the marginal branch of the circumflex artery (2). Two venous bypasses to the affected vessels are present; one to the anterior interventricular artery (+), the other to the circumflex artery (o). Note the sternotomy, with streak artefacts arising from the presence of a metallic clip.

Film obtained without i.v. contrast.

b Both venous grafts (→) are patent, as shown by the opacification simultaneously with the aorta, 12 s after a rapid i.v. bolus injection of 60 ml 76% iodine dye. The pulmonary arterial trunk (pt) is already drained of its contrast medium, but the left pulmonary veins (pv) are still densely opacified

Fig. 4.77. Double aortocoronary vein bypass. The grafts are to the right coronary artery (►) and to the anterior interventricular artery (▷), easily identified in the rich mediastinal fat. Both grafts are proved to be patent by their opacification up to 241 HU after rapid i.v. bolus injection of contrast medium. Note the opacification of the internal mammary arteries (→)

Fig. 4.78. Triple aortocoronary graft. While the two grafts to the anterior interventricular artery (▷) and to the circumflex artery (→) are patent, the density inside the right coronary artery bypass (►) during the passage of the rapid iodine bolus does not exceed 83 HU, which indicates lack of patency. Note the opacification of the main trunk of the original left coronary artery (⇨)

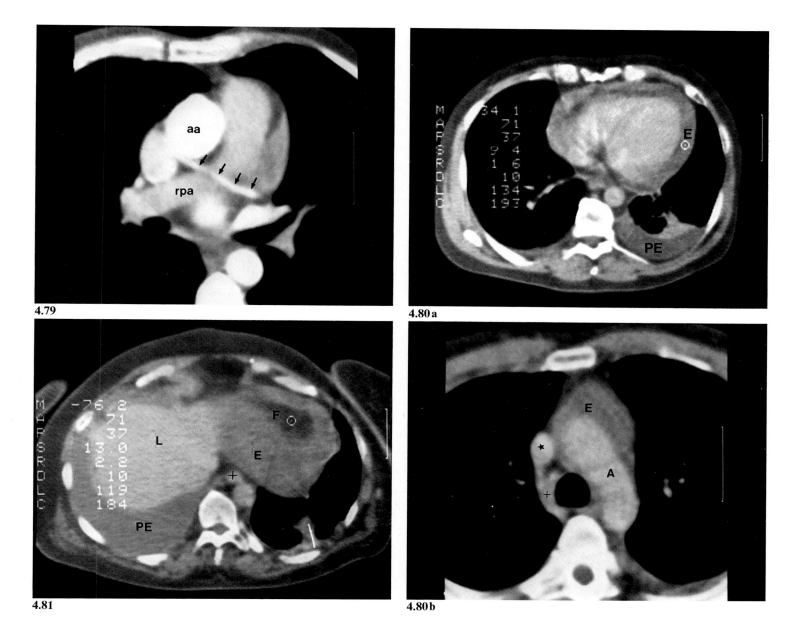

4.79　**4.80 a**

4.81　**4.80 b**

Fig. 4.79. Venous aortocoronary bypass to the circumflex artery (→). This graft is shown in its typical horizontal position, crossing posterior to the ascending aorta (*aa*) and below the right pulmonary artery (*rpa*) within the transverse pericardial sinus from the right lateral aortic wall to the left coronary sulcus. This bypass proves to be patent, as indicated by its opacification, which is as great as that of the aorta during the first passage of the rapid i.v. bolus of contrast. The remaining two grafts in this patient are not opacified, and are consequently occluded

Pericardium

Fig. 4.80 a, b. Pericardial effusion. **a** The effusion (*E*) surrounds the ventricular mass of the heart. The elevated density of the fluid accumulation (34 HU) strongly suggests a haemorrhagic effusion. In addition, a left basal pleural effusion (*PE*) and pulmonary hypoventilation are present. Intravenous contrast injection more clearly defines the pericardial accumulation, especially when the density of the haemorrhagic component equals that of the myocardium. **b** The pericardial accumulation (*E*) extends anteriorly as high as the aortic arch (*A*). At that level the azygos vein (+) crosses anteriorly to join the superior vena cava (★).

Films obtained after i.v. contrast administration

Fig. 4.81. Pericardial effusion. A very specific sign showing a fluid collection to be of pericardial origin is the demonstration of the epicardial fat (*F*) inside the collection. This is particularly helpful in differentiating pericardial effusion at the level of the diaphragm from pleural fluid or subphrenic collections. *E*, pericardial effusion; *PE*, pleural effusion; *L*, liver; +, oesophagus.

For a reconstruction display of a pericardial collection in the coronary plane, see Fig. 4.57 b

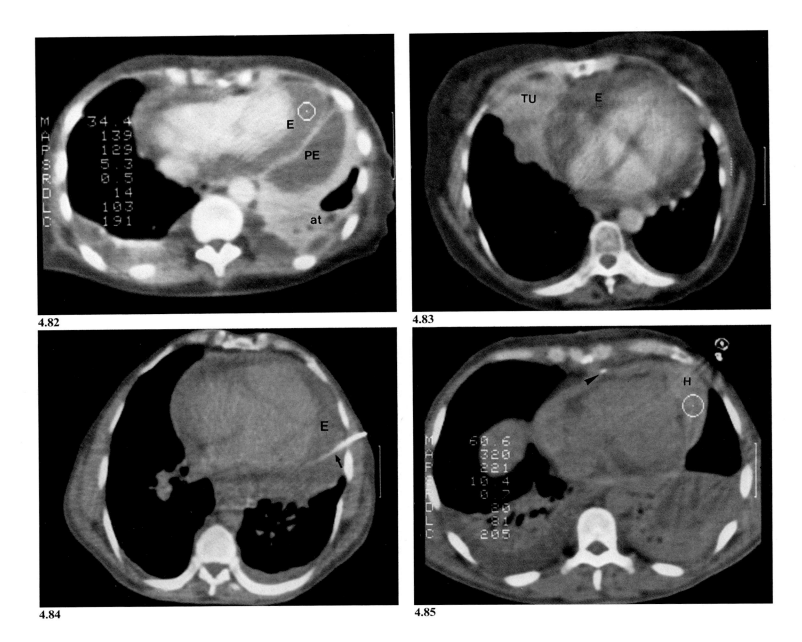

4.82

4.83

4.84

4.85

Fig. 4.82. Haemorrhagic pericardial effusion. The effusion (*E*) is accompanied by a pleural empyema (*PE*). In these circumstances CT is more sensitive than ultrasound for the detection of pericardial accumulations. It may be impossible to differentiate empyema fluid from a haemorrhagic collection; however, densities higher than 30 HU are more likely to represent a haemorrhagic effusion. There is left inferior lobe atelectasis (*at*).

Film obtained after i.v. bolus injection

Fig. 4.84. CT-guided drainage of a pericardial effusion. In this patient the usual subxyphoid puncture for pericardial fluid drainage was unsuccessful. The CT examination which was thus performed indicated that the left laterothoracic approach would be best for the pericardial puncture: 300 ml haemorrhagic fluid were subsequently aspirated. A 16-gauge plastic catheter is in place (→). No i.v. contrast injection

Fig. 4.83. Pericardial effusion in a case of malignant thymoma. The effusion (*E*) is due to tumour invasion (*Tu*), which extends into the anterior parietal and the mediastinal pleura, as well as the pericardium.

Film obtained late after i.v. contrast administration

Fig. 4.85. Cardiac tamponade. A high-density (over 60 HU) accumulation is present within the pericardial sac, corresponding to a recent postoperative haemorrhage (*H*). The blood is clotted with haemoconcentration, which explains the elevated density. This patient had had resection of a ventricular aneurysm and showed clinical signs of cardiac tamponade in the days after operation.
Bilateral basal pleural effusions with partial atelectases are present. A postoperative drainage tube is seen in the anterior mediastinum (►).

Image not contrast enhanced

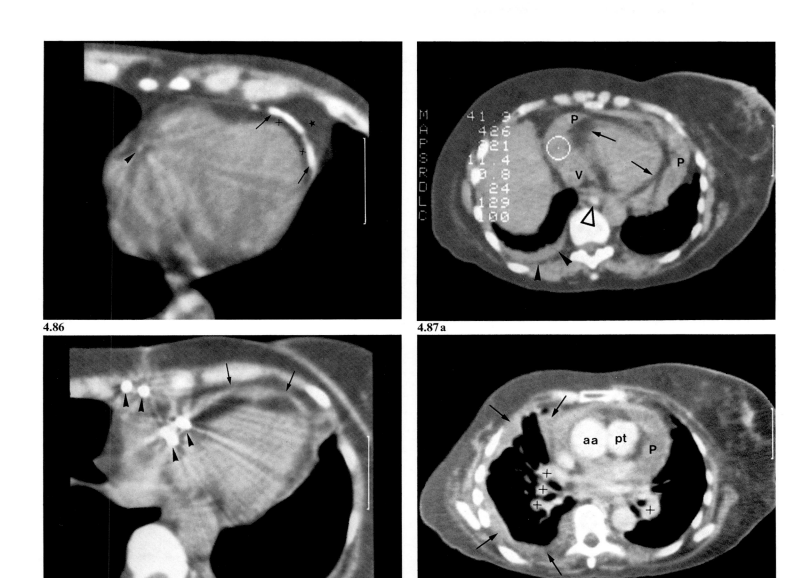

4.86

4.87a

4.88

4.87b

Fig. 4.86. Pericardial calcification. Note that the pericardium separates the epicardial fat (+) from the pericardial fat (★). A slightly calcified right coronary artery (►) is the source of the multiple streak artefacts. The patient's history suggests that the pericardial calcification (→) is of a tubercular origin.

No contrast injection

Fig. 4.88. Postoperative pericardial thickening. The thickening (→) is due to the recent implantation of an epicardial pacemaker (►).

No contrast administration

Fig. 4.87a, b. Constrictive fibrous pericarditis of tumoral origin. **a** There is a circumferential homogeneous pericardial thickening up to 2 cm in diameter, whose density is about 40 HU. Furthermore, the right diaphragm is elevated and the right posterior pleura (►) is thickened.
The epicardial fat layer (→) separates the fibrous pericardium (P) from the heart muscle. The oesophagus (▷) is filled with Gastrografin (meglumine diatrizoate). The inferior vena cava (V) is widened, indicating right heart failure.
Note the absence of the right breast due to mastectomy for cancer, followed by radiotherapy.

Film obtained without contrast injection

b At the level of the aortic (aa) and pulmonary (pt) roots, there is extensive parietal and mediastinal pleural thickening (→). The enlarged pulmonary veins (+) indicate pulmonary congestion due to left heart failure.
The pericardium (P) enhanced very slightly from 40 HU to 50 HU after i.v. bolus injection. Pericardial carcinomatosis was diagnosed at autopsy

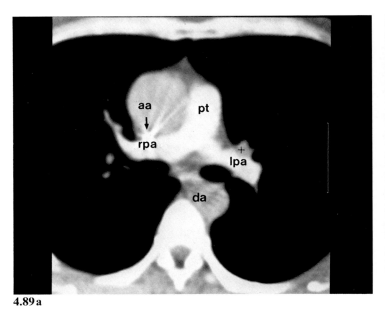

4.89 a

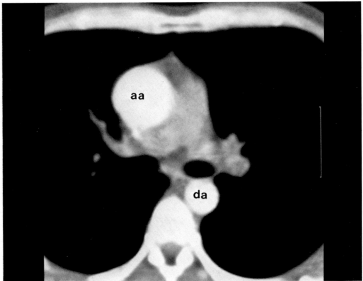

4.89 b

Great Thoracic Arteries

Fig. 4.89 a, b. Selective opacification of normal pulmonary arteries. **a** The pulmonary trunk (*pt*), right pulmonary artery (*rpa*) and left pulmonary artery (*lpa*) are opacified. The almost undiluted contrast material within the superior vena cava (→) causes streak artefacts. Note that the ascending (*aa*) and descending (*da*) aorta and the left superior pulmonary vein (+) are not yet filled with dye.

The technique used was rapid bolus injection within 3 s of 60 ml 76% iodine dye into a cubital vein with a 16-gauge needle. The film was exposed during the 5 s immediately following injection, corresponding to a normal circulation time.

b Selective opacification of the ascending and descending aorta in the same patient. The iodine bolus is now passing almost selectively through the thoracic aorta, while the pulmonary arterial tree is perfused by unopacified blood. There is a mild degree of ectasia of the ascending aorta (diameter 4.5 cm).

This image is the second of a series taken after rapid bolus injection, starting 10 s after the exposure described in **a**, i.e. 15 s after the bolus injection

Fig. 4.90. Pneumomediastinum of the periaortic space. The arciform airshadow (→) surrounding the left lateral wall of the descending aorta (*da*) is pathognomonic for a pneumomediastinum, which is best seen with a window width above 1,000 HU. Anteriorly an additional small pneumopericardium (►) is present in this polytraumatized patient

Fig. 4.91. Right aortic arch and aberrant left subclavian artery. The air-filled oesophagus (→) is situated between the trachea and the

slightly calcified aberrant left subclavian artery (+). The aortic arch (*AA*) is located to the right of the trachea. The patient began to get dysphagia when 50 years old, by which time sclerotic arterial changes had led to compression of the oesophagus.

No contrast injection

Fig. 4.92. Aortic diverticulum. At the level of the aortic arch (*AA*) is a retrotracheal pouch with arterial opacification and a large neck towards the posterior medial part of the aortic arch. In this asymptomatic young (29-year-old) man this finding is consistent with a congenital aortic diverticulum (*AD*). *VC*, superior vena cava.

Scan obtained after rapid i.v. bolus injection

Fig. 4.93. Marfan's syndrome. Note the elongated and tortuous aortic arch (*AA*) and the absence of arteriosclerotic calcifications. The superior vena cava (+) is also to be seen. This is the same patient as in Fig. 4.74.

Film obtained late after i.v. contrast injection

Fig. 4.94. Pulmonary hypertension. This 16-year-old girl with combined mitral failure, predominant mitral insufficiency and pulmonary hypertension (already discussed in Fig. 4.54) had a mitral valve prosthesis. The pulmonary trunk (*pt*) is dilated to 37 mm in diameter, which is striking in comparison with the relatively small ascending aorta (*aa*). Note the operation scar in the anterior mediastinum (★) and the mild widening of the superior vena cava (*svc*).

Picture obtained after bolus injection

104

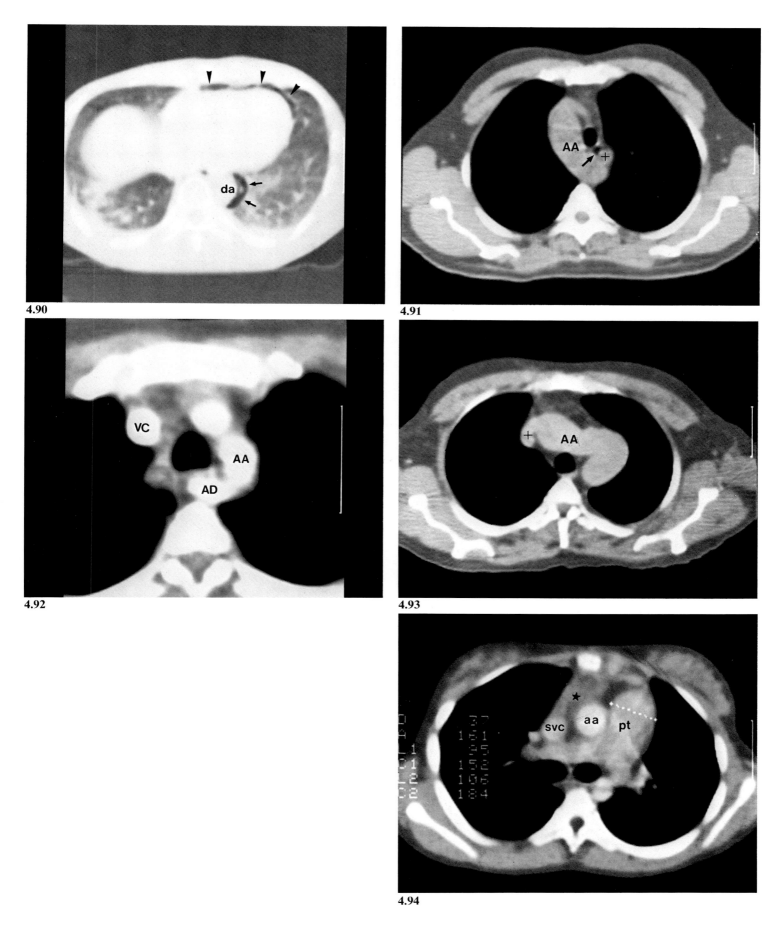

4.90

4.91

4.92

4.93

4.94

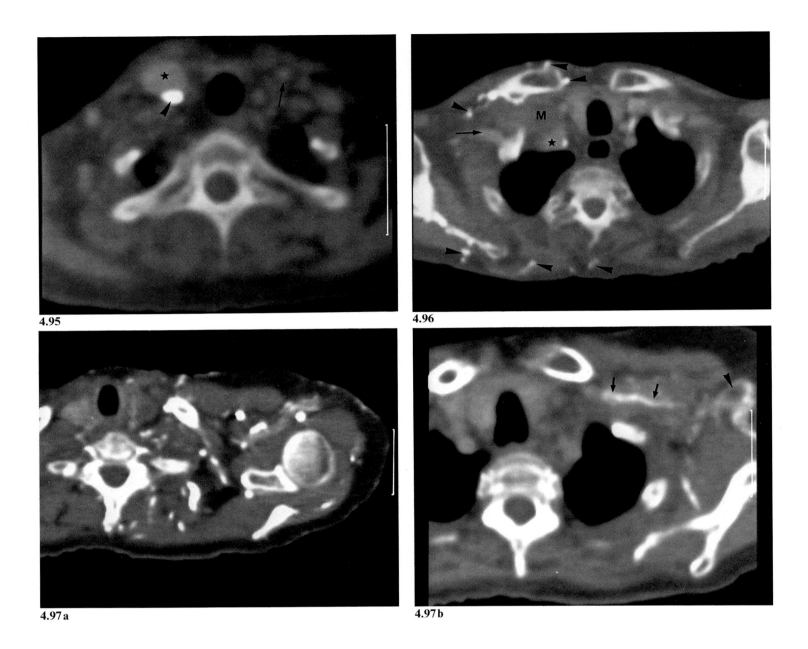

4.95

4.96

4.97 a

4.97 b

Great Thoracic Veins

Fig. 4.95. Physiological asymmetry of the internal jugular veins. The right internal jugular vein (★) is 2 cm in diameter, but the left one (→) does not exceed 5 mm. The right subclavian vein (►), filled with the iodine bolus, enters the jugular vein at this level. The patient was studied because of the presence of a right laterocervical mass, which was due entirely to the enlarged internal jugular vein.

Film obtained after bolus injection into a right cubital vein

Fig. 4.96. Tumoral compression. Compression is being exerted by a retroclavicular metastasis (*M*) at the confluence of the right subclavian vein (→) and the jugular vein (★). The collateral subcutaneous

veins (►) are filled in the anterior chest wall and in the periscapular region.

Film obtained after right cubital vein bolus injection

Fig. 4.97a, b. Brachiocephalic vein thrombosis. **a** There are collateral veins in the left upper thoracic region due to the thrombosis. The cutaneous, periscapular and paravertebral dilated veins are densely filled after left cubital bolus injection. **b** The left subclavian vein (→) presents a reduced and irregular lumen and is surrounded by soft tissue swelling, consistent with thrombophlebitic changes. A central filling defect present in the left axillary vein (►), consistent with thrombosis, is barely enveloped by contrast material

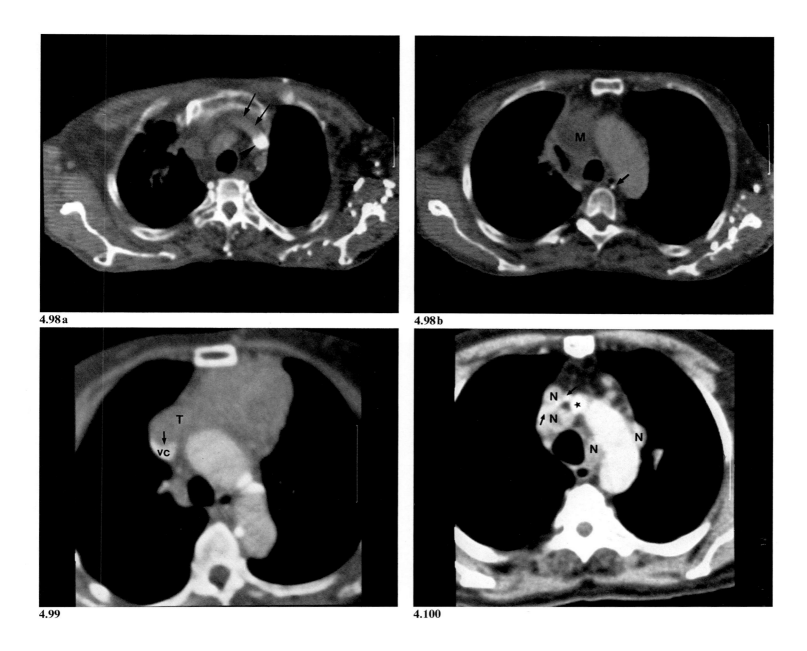

4.98a

4.98b

4.99

4.100

Fig. 4.98a, b. Tumoral occlusion of the left brachiocephalic vein and superior vena cava by an underlying mediastinal lymph node metastasis from a pulmonary carcinoma. a The site of the left brachiocephalic occlusion is demonstrated by the obliteration of the brachiocephalic vein (→) medially and by the dense retained head of the i.v. bolus (▶) laterally. Venous drainage is achieved by multiple subcutaneous, periscapular and perivertebral veins. b The superior vena cava is also occluded by the metastasis (M). Venous drainage is effected by the left periscapular venous plexus and by an accessory hemiazygos vein (→) which is situated posterior to the oesophagus.

Film obtained early after left cubital bolus injection

Fig. 4.99. Tumour invasion of the superior vena cava by a malignant thymoma. A bulging tumour mass (T) in the anterior mediastinum penetrates anteriorly (→) into the lumen of the strongly deformed superior vena cava (VC). The i.v. contrast material opacifies the residual lumen of the vena cava and the calcified aortic arch

Fig. 4.100. Compression of the superior vena cava. Two metastatic lymphnodes (N) situated in front of and posterior to the superior vena cava (→) cause a considerable stenosis by compression. Other nodes are seen on either side of the aortic arch. The origin of the brachiocephalic artery (★) is visible.

Film obtained after i.v. bolus injection

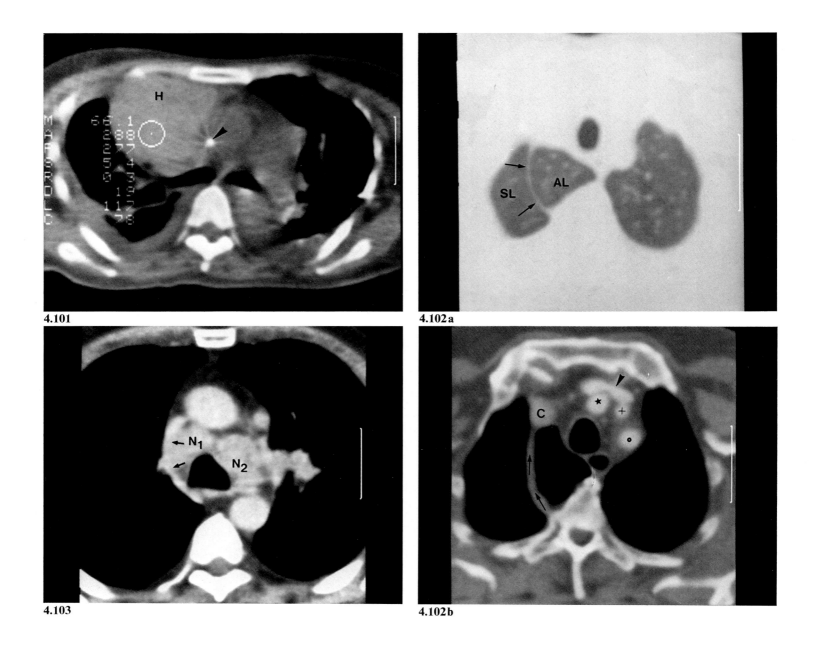

4.101

4.102 a

4.103

4.102 b

Fig. 4.101. Large iatrogenic mediastinal haematoma. The fresh hae-matoma (*H*) is due to the positioning of a catheter in the right subcla-vian vein and has a density of 66 HU. The opaque venous catheter (▶) is visualized within the superior vena cava, which is compressed by the haematoma.

No contrast injection

Fig. 4.103. Deviation of the azygos vein (→) by a metastatic lymph A node (*N₁*). A second node (*N₂*) is situated in the aortic window. This is the patient already discussed in Fig. 4.101.

Film obtained after i.v. contrast injection

Fig. 4.102. a Accessory azygos lobe. The accessory lobe (*AL*) is sepa-rated by a thin pleural septum (→) from the remaining part of the right superior lobe (*SL*). **b** Intrapulmonary cross of the azygos vein (→) in the same patient at a slightly lower level. The cross section demonstrates the superior vena cava (*C*), the brachiocephalic artery (★), the left common carotid artery (+), the left subclavian artery (o) and in transverse section the left innominate vein (▶).

Film obtained after left cubital i.v. bolus injection

108

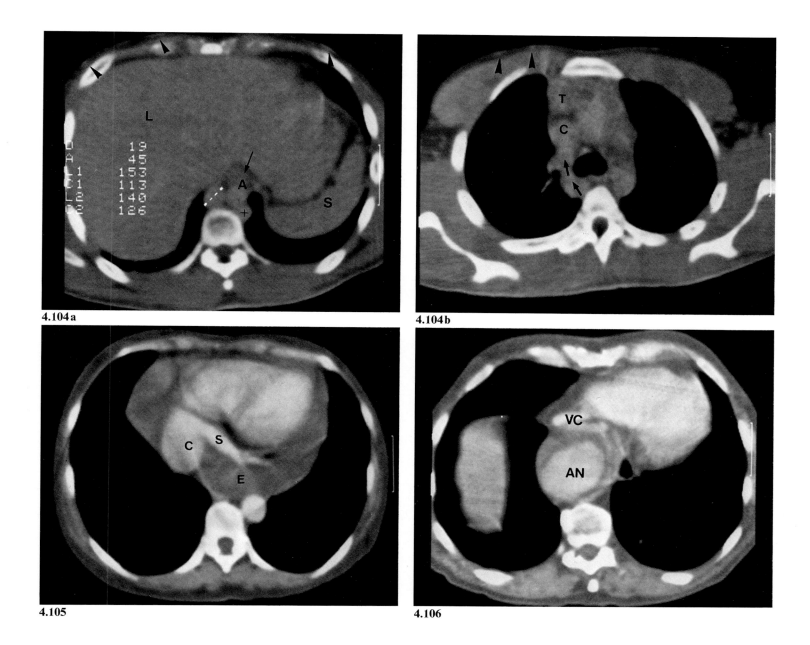

4.104 a

4.104 b

4.105

4.106

Fig. 4.104a, b. Azygos and hemiazygos vein continuation in the lower mediastinum due to inferior vena cava obstruction by a retroperitoneal tumour. **a** The enlarged azygos vein (19 mm in diameter) is situated to the right of the descending aorta (*A*), the similarly dilated hemiazygos vein (+) to its left. The cardio-oesophageal junction (→) is located in front of the aorta. Note the enlarged cutaneous veins (►) of the anterior chest wall and the absence of the inferior vena cava. *L*, liver; *S*, spleen.

Film obtained late after i.v. contrast injection.

b In the same patient there is widening of the azygos vein at its cross (→) entering the superior vena cava (*C*). An anterior mediastinal tumour is also present (*T*), and the subcutaneous collateral veins (►) are visible.

Film obtained late after i.v. contrast injection

Fig. 4.105. Inferior vena cava enlargement. The enlargement is due to right heart failure in a case of mitral disease and large pericardial effusion (*E*). The coronary sinus (*S*) enters the widened inferior vena cava (*C*). This is the same patient as in Fig. 4.68.

Film obtained after i.v. bolus injection

Fig. 4.106. Inferior vena cava compression by a partially thrombosed descending aortic aneurysm. The inferior vena cava (*VC*) is significantly compressed and displaced anteriorly by the aneurysm (*AN*).

Film obtained after i.v. bolus injection

109

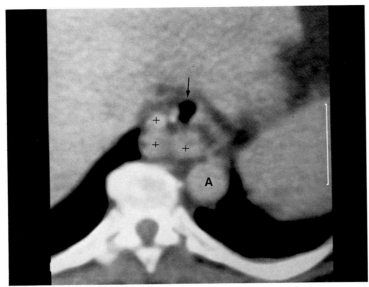

4.107

Fig. 4.107. Perioesophageal varices due to liver cirrhosis. The nodular opacities (+) in the lower mediastinum, interposed between the lower oesophagus (→), the descending aorta (A) and the vertebral body, have densities equal to that of the aorta and are consistent with large varicose nodes (20 mm in diameter).

Film obtained late after i.v. contrast injection

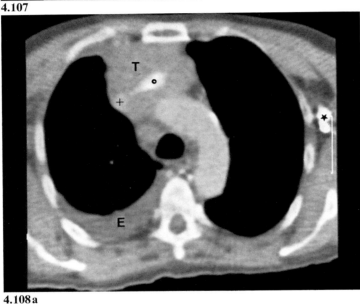

4.108 a

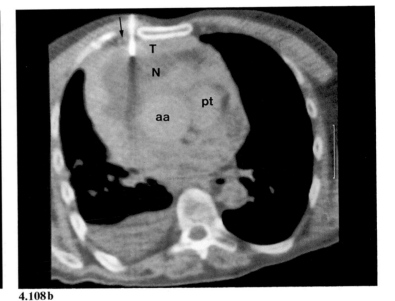

4.108 b

An Anatomopathological Correlation with CT in One Patient

Fig. 4.108 a, b. Superior vena cava compression by a large anterior mediastinal tumour of unknown nature. **a** The 67-year-old patient had progressive bilateral jugular vein stasis. A solid invasive tumour (T) causes compression at the confluence of the right (+) and left (o) brachiocephalic veins. The i.v. bolus is retained in the left axillary vein (★). In addition, a right pleural effusion is present (E). CT diagnosis at this point includes the differential diagnosis of a malignant solid tumour: thymoma, mesothelioma, histiocytoma, lymphoma, metastasis of an unknown primary tumour. **b** Anterior parasternal CT-guided mediastinal biopsy (with a tru-cut needle). The upper thoracic venous stasis represented a contra-indication to mediastinoscopy; for this reason a needle biopsy was chosen, so that the treatment could be based on a histological diagnosis. The needle enters the free window between the sternum and the right internal mammary vessels (→) and penetrates 1 cm into the tumoral tissue (T), remaining at a safe distance from the ascending aorta (aa) and the pulmonary trunk (pt). The superior vena cava is obliterated. The neoplasm invades the pericardium and the anterior aortic wall and surrounds the mediastinal structures completely. Note the hypodense centre of the mass, probably due to necrosis (N).

The biopsy material was of a good quality, and no postbiopsy complications occurred. Histopathological analysis led to a diagnosis of fibrous mesothelioma (probable) or histiocytoma with no certain malignancy (possible). Palliative radiotherapy treatment led to clinical improvement and regression of the venous stasis

110

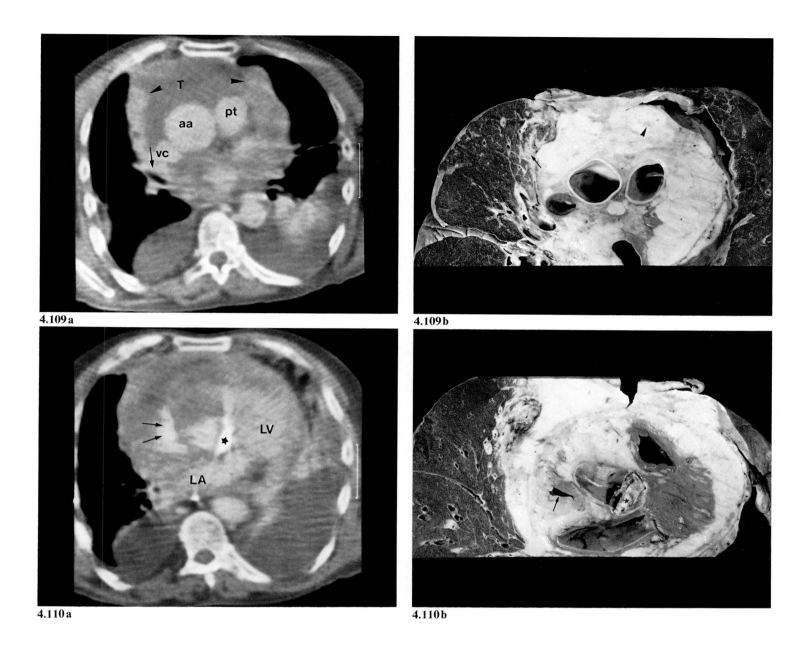

4.109a

4.109b

4.110a

4.110b

Fig. 4.109a, b. Because of progressive cardiac failure, a control study was carried out 5 weeks after biopsy to search for a pericardial effusion. The patient died a few days later. At autopsy 1-cm-thick thoracic cross sections were obtained for correlation with the CT study. The definitive histopathological diagnosis, was malignant fibrous mesothelioma of the pericardium. **a** CT cross section at the level of the aortic (*aa*) and pulmonary (*pt*) roots. The superior vena cava (*vc*) is moderately narrowed. The tumour (*T*) consists of a thick, nodular outer wall (►) and a hypodense inner shell surrounding all the mediastinal structures like a ring. There is invasion and compression of the right main bronchus (→). **b** Anatomopathological cross section at the same level. Extensive tumoral invasion of the whole mediastinum. The hypodense centre of the tumour is due to fatty degeneration

(►), probably following radiotherapy. The crater-like stenosis of the superior vena cava is clearly evident.

In addition, tumour invasion of the pulmonary parenchyma is seen in the right anterior paramediastinal region (→)

Fig. 4.110. a CT at the level of the supravalvular aorta shows a large calcified plaque (★) of the medial wall. The superior vena cava is grossly stenosed (→). The roof of the left ventricle (*LV*) is in contact with the tumoral tissue, as is the upper part of the left atrium (*LA*). There are bilateral pleural effusions. **b** The corresponding anatomopathological cross section shows extensive tumoral encasement of all vascular structures, in particular of the superior vena cava (→). The calcified aortic plaque (★) is also seen

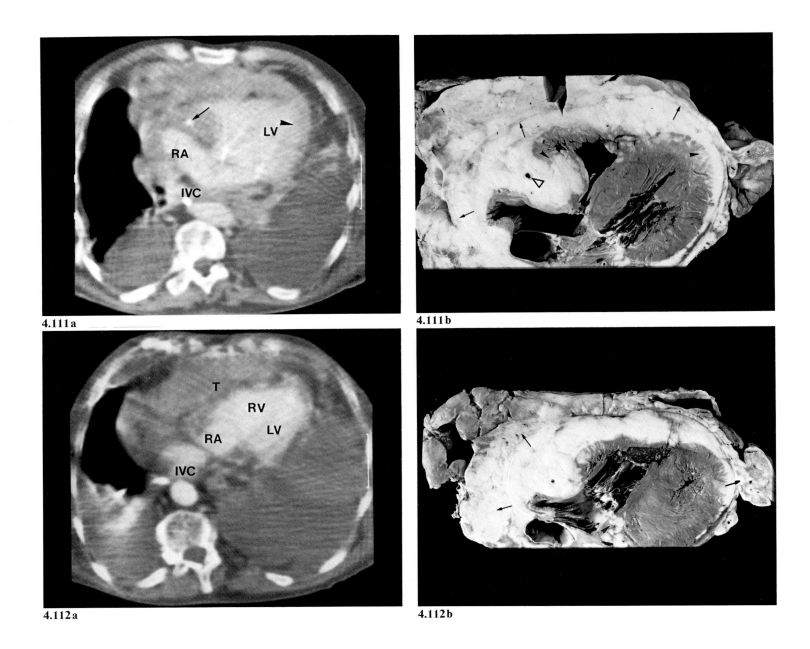

4.111a

4.111b

4.112a

4.112b

Fig. 4.111. a At the level of the left ventricle (*LV*) extensive tumoral invasion of the right coronary sulcus can be seen, with the calcified coronary artery at its centre (→). The right atrium (*RA*) is separated from the inferior vena cava (*IVC*). Note the absence of epicardial fat at the lateral wall (►) of the left ventricle, where no delimitation of the tumour towards the myocardium is possible. **b** In spite of the massive extent of the tumour, the pericardial wall is still recognizable (→). The tumour deeply invades the right coronary sulcus with the coronary artery (▷) at its centre. In several areas there is tumoral infiltration of the myocardium (►). No space is left for a pericardial fluid collection

Fig. 4.112. a Cross section through the base of the heart showing the right (*RV*) and left (*LV*) ventricles, the right atrium (*RA*) and the inferior vena cava (*IVC*). The lower anterior mediastinum is still occupied by a thick layer of tumoral tissue (*T*). **b** Cross section through the tricuspid valve and the apex of the left ventricle. Tumoral nodules (►) are seen in the inferior posterior part of the septum. The visible pericardial fat shows severe tumoral infiltration (→)

The anatomopathological cross sections in Figs. 4.108–4.112 are courtesy of Dr. L. Vavassori, Department of Pathology, and Professor Kapanci, Chief of the Clinical Division, University Hospital, Geneva, Switzerland.

4.4 Aneurysms of the Thoracic Aorta

N. Vasile, D. Larde, and J. Ferrané

CT is most valuable in the evaluation of known or presumed mediastinal masses, allowing differentiation between vascular and non-vascular structures. The introduction of contrast injection (angio CT) adds a new dimension, permitting the recognition of lumen patency or mural thrombus and facilitating the diagnosis of dissecting aneurysms. Another possible use of this non-invasive procedure is the follow-up of small aneurysms in routine postoperative evaluation of patients.

4.4.1 Technique

All examination should be performed on third-generation machine with a scan time under 5 s. The initial scan is obtained without contrast medium in order to determine the area of interest. Bolus injection of up to 40 ml contrast material is then performed, followed immediately by scans of the previously defined area. The injection is repeated in each area, up to a total of about 2 ml iodine/kg body weight.

4.4.2 Semiology

Aneurysms of the thoracic aorta have five characteristics:
1. Localized dilatation of the aorta, whose lumen is more than 4 cm in diameter (Cooley)
2. Curvilinear and plaque-like intimal calcifications at the edge of the aorta, detected more sensitively than by conventional radiography and well located on a cross-sectional view
3. Loss of parallelism of the borders of the horizontal aorta

4. A laminated or circular intraluminal thrombus
5. Displacement of the mediastinal structures

In traumatic aneurysms, CT can reveal haematoma in continuity with the aorta, or pleural fluid. It is a safe method for exploring the mediastinum and seeking abdominal or vertebral lesions in severely injured patients.

In all cases, anatomical localization on the aorta is easy and vertical extension into the abdomen can be studied. Two differential diagnoses can be considered:
1. Juxta-aortic tumour (but in this case the structure is frequently heterogeneous and the density increases more slowly than in vascular lumen
2. Plain tortuous atherosclerotic aorta or aortic kinking

The diagnosis of dissecting aortic aneurysms relies on four findings:
1. Localized increase of aortic calibre (the only constant finding)
2. The presence of displaced intimal calcifications
3. The existence of an intimal flap separating the true and false channels
4. Confirmation of a false channel whose lumen is less dense because of the slower flow rate

Theoretically, dissection can be differentiated from aneurysm of the aorta by the presence of displaced intimal calcifications and by the detection of an intimal flap. The only real difficulty in diagnosis comes when a completely occluded false channel has the some low density as an aneurysm with a peripheral thrombus.

Postoperatively, CT can reveal an increase in the size of the aorta at the site of vascular graft (false aneurysm) and can also show infection.

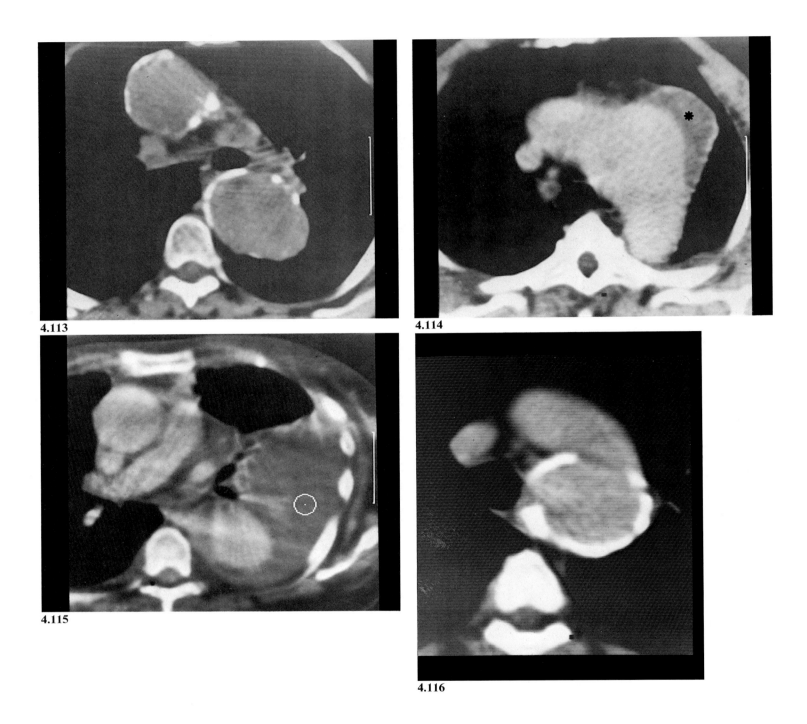

4.113

4.114

4.115

4.116

Fig. 4.113. Local dilatation of the thoracic aorta. The diameter of the ascending aorta is 5 cm, of the descending aorta 6,3 cm. Note the plaque-like intimal calcifications at the edge of the aorta and the syphilitic aneurysm of the arch [17]

Fig. 4.115. Blunt chest trauma. The aorta, opacified by contrast material, is clearly visible. There is a haemothorax and a haematoma surrounding the descending aorta [14]

Fig. 4.114. Intraluminal thrombus. A CT scan with contrast infusion shows loss of parallelism of the walls of the horizontal aorta with an increase in diameter, revealing the thrombus (*). Contrast material fills the patent portion of the lumen

Fig. 4.116. Huge calcified aneurysm of isthmic aorta

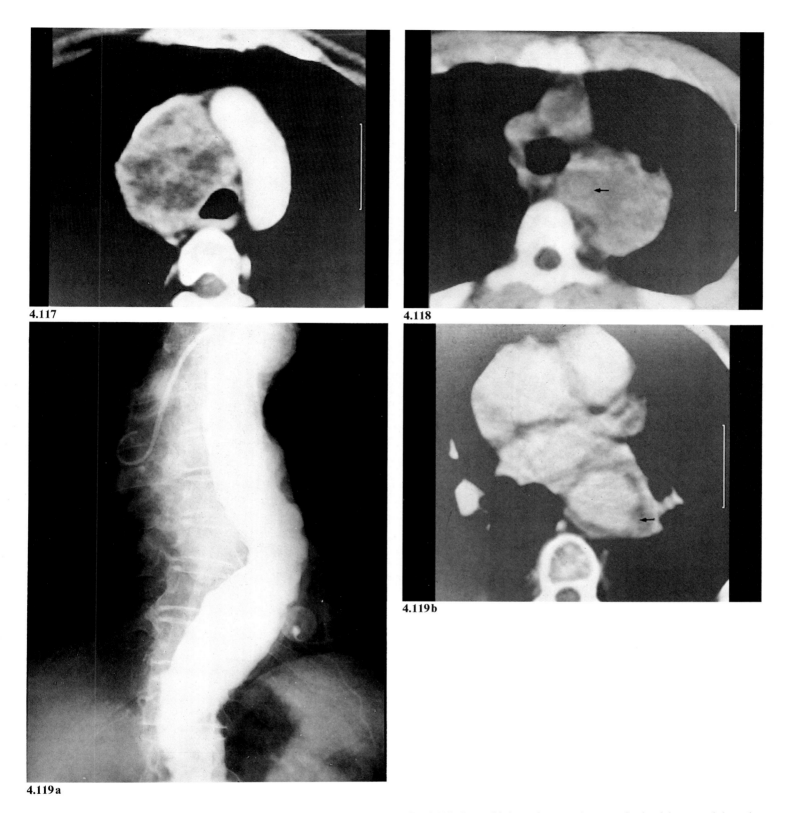

4.117

4.118

4.119b

4.119a

Fig. 4.118. Bronchial carcinoma. A scan obtained just caudal to the aortic arch without intravenous administration of contrast medium, shows the carcinoma surrounding the descending aorta (←)

Fig. 4.117. Juxta-aortic bronchial carcinoma. CT with contrast infusion reveals the tumour, which simulated an aortic aneurysm on plain films. The vascular lumen is opacified. The tumour is heterogeneous, with central hypodensity corresponding to necrosis

Fig. 4.119. a An aortogram shows atheromatous irregularities of the descending aorta without aneurysm. b A contrast-enhanced scan points out the same irregularities with a non-opacified mural thrombus (←)

115

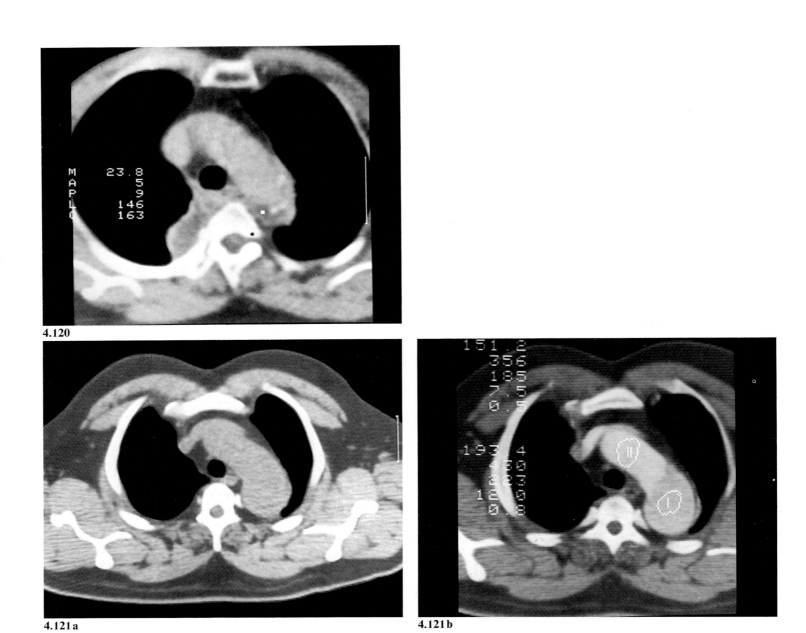

4.120

4.121 a

4.121 b

Fig. 4.120. CT before contrast injection in the descending aorta reveals that the wall is thickened and the intimal calcifications are displaced inwards, indicating dissection [20, 47]

Fig. 4.121. a Before contrast injection the descending aorta is slightly dilated. **b** CT scans taken within 30 s of the bolus injection of contrast medium show that the false channel has a lower density (150 HU) than the aortic lumen (193 HU) because of the different flow rates in the two channels. Note the mediastinal lipomatosis adjacent to the outside of the anterolateral wall of the aortic arch, and also the false impression of dissection created by the course of the left brachiocephalic vein anterior to the aortic arch

116

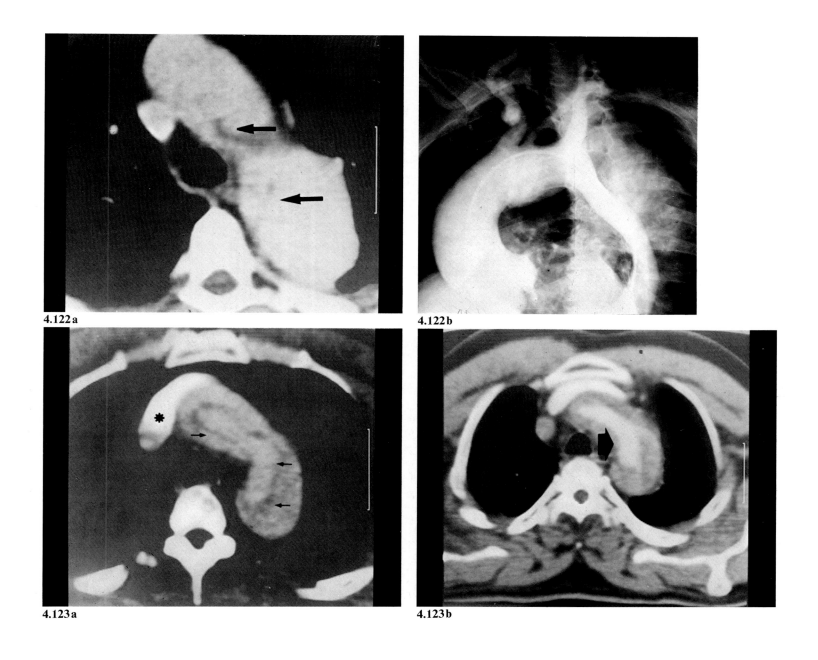

4.122 a

4.122 b

4.123 a

4.123 b

Fig. 4.123a, b. Intimal flap. Scans obtained at aortic arch level. **a** A few seconds after bolus injection, contrast medium opacifies the superior vena cava (∗). The intimal flap is a radiolucent crescent shown medially in the aortic arch (→). **b** At 30 s there is an enhanced true lumen (◖) with discrete enhancement of the false lumen

Fig. 4.122. a Intimal flap (←). **b** Aortogram shows a type III dissection with a non-opacified false lumen compressing the true lumen. No intimal flap is seen

117

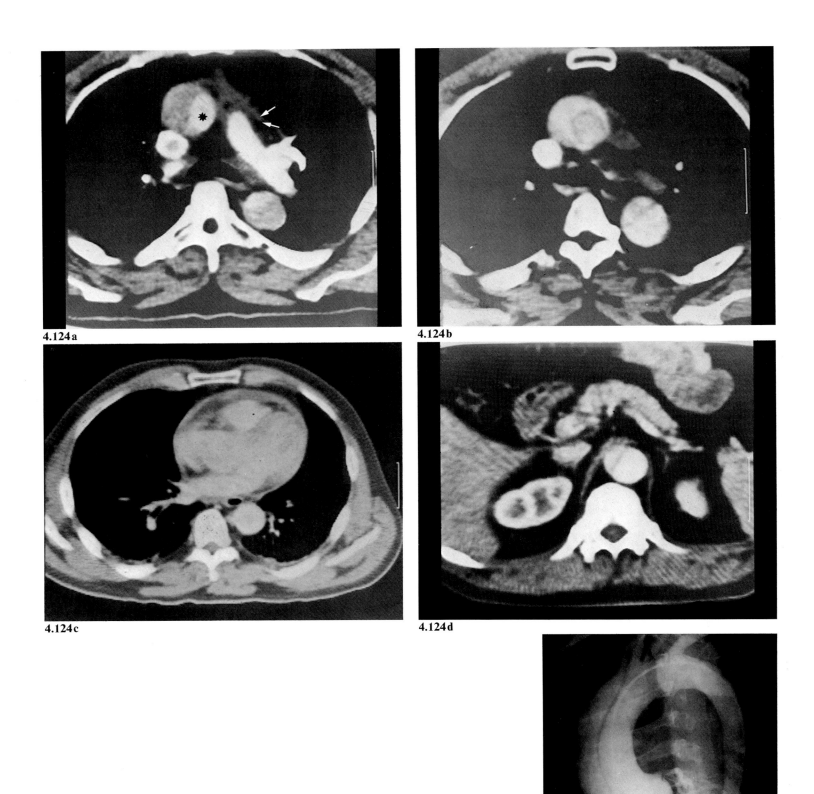

4.124a

4.124b

4.124c

4.124d

Fig. 4.124. a CT scan 15 s after contrast bolus. The left pulmonary artery is contrast enhanced (←) and the true lumen is opacified (∗). **b** At 30 s, a scan taken 1 cm higher shows an intimal flap in the ascending and descending aorta. **c** Pericardial effusion. **d** The intimal flap extends to the abdominal aorta. **e** Control aortogram. The ascending aorta is dilated, and the intimal flap is seen; there is an aortic insufficiency

4.124e

References

1. Adams DF, Hessel SJ, Judy PF, Stein JA, Abrams HL (1976) Computed tomography of the normal and infarcted myocardium. Comput Tomogr 126(4):786–791
2. Aita JF, Wanamaker WM (1979) Body computerized tomography and the thymus. Arch Neurol 36:30–21
3. Belloir C, Lardé D, Vasile N, Frija J, Ferrané J (1980) Apport de la tomodensitométrie dans le diagnostic et le bilan des anévrysmes de l'aorte. J Radiol 61:521–526
4. Berninger WH, Redington, RW, Doherty P, Lipton MJ, Carlsson E (1979) Gated cardiac scanning: canine studies. J Comput Assist Tomogr 3(2):155–163
5. Binder RE, Pugatch RD, Faling LJ, Kanter RA, Sawin CT (1980) Diagnosis of posterior mediastinal goiter by computed tomography. J Comput Assist Tomogr 4:550–552
6. Blin ME, Mancuso AA, Mink JH, Hansen BC (1978) Computed tomography in the evaluation of mediastinal lipomatosis. J Comput Assist Tomogr 2:375–383
7. Carlsson E, Lipton MJ, Skiöldebrand CG, Berninger WH, Redinc RW (1980) Erfahrungen mit der Computer-Tomographie bei der in vivo-Herzdiagnostik. Radiologe 20:44–49
8. Carter BL, Ignatow SB (1977) Neck and mediastinal angiography by computed tomography scan. Radiology 122:515–516
9. Coulomb M, Dyon JF, Labas JF, Sarrazin R (1979) Aspects normaux et variations non pathologiques en tomodensitométrie du médiastin chez l'adulte. J Radiol 60:463–476
11. Crowe JK, Brown LR, Muhm JR (1978) Computed tomography of the mediastinum. Radiology 128:75–88
12. Daffner RH, Halber MD, Postlethwait RW, Korobkin M, Thompson WM (1979) C.T. of the esophagus II. Carcinoma. AJR 133:1051–1055
13. Doppman JL, Rienmuller R, Lissner J, Cyran J, Bolte HD, Strauer BE, Hellwig H (1981) Computed tomography in constrictive pericardial disease. J Comput Assist Tomogr 5(1):1–11
14. Egan TJ, Neiman HL, Herman RJ, Malave SR, Sanders JH (1980) Computed tomography in the diagnosis of aortic aneurysm dissection or traumatic injury. Radiology 136:141–146
15. Emami B, Melo A, Carter BL, Munzenrider JE, Piro AJ (1978) The value of computed tomography in radiotherapy of lung cancer. AJR 131:63–68
16. Ferrane J, Utzmann O, Le Cudonnec B, Vasile N (1979) Tomodensitométrie cardiaque. Anatomie normale. J Radiol 60(3):169–173
17. Godwin JD, Herfkens RJ, Skioldebrand CG, Federle MP, Lipton MJ (1980) Evaluation of dissections and aneurysms of the thoracic aorta by conventional and dynamic CT scanning. Radiology 136:125–133
18. Godwin JD, Turley K, Herfkens RJ, Lipton MJ (1981) Computed tomography for follow-up of chronic aortic dissections. Radiology 139:655
19. Goldwin RL, Heitzman ER, Prato AV (1977) Computed tomography of the mediastinum normal anatomy and indications for the use of C.T. Radiology 124:235–241
20. Gross SC, Barr I, Eyler WR, Khaja F, Goldstein S (1980) Computed tomography in dissection of the thoracic aorta. Radiology 136:135–139
21. Guthaner GF, Miller DC, Silverman JF, Stinson EB, Wexler L (1979) Fate of the false lumen following surgical repair of aortic dissections: angiographic study. Radiology 133:1
22. Guthaner DF, Wexler L, Harell G (1979) CT demonstration of cardiac structures. AJR 133:75–81
23. Guthaner DF, Brody WR, Ricci M, Oyer PE, Wexler L (1980) The use of computed tomography in the diagnosis of coronary artery bypass graft patency. Cardiovasc Intervent Radiol 3:3–8
24. Halber MD (1980) C.T. of esophagus. Incorrect labeling. Reply. AJR 135:425
25. Haller DM, Daffner RH, Thompson WM (1979) C.T. of the oesophagus; normal appearance. AJR 133:1047–1055
26. Hauser H (1980) Tomométrie axiale cardiaque. Méd Hyg 38:2192–2194
27. Hauser H, Perrenoud JJ, Bopp P, Rutishauser W, Hahn C (1980) La tomoradiométrie transverse dans le contrôle de la perméabilité des ponts aorto-coronariens: valeur et intérêt par rapport à la coronarographie. Schweiz Med Wochenschr 110(45):1651–1654
28. Heiberg E, Wolvarson MK, Sundaram M (1981) CT Finding in thoracic dissection. AJR 136:13
29. Heitzman ER (1977) The mediastinum, radiologic correlations with anatomy and pathology. C.V. Mosby, St Louis
30. Heitzmann ER (1981) Computed tomography of the thorax: current perspectives. AJR 136:2–12
31. Heitzman ER, Goldwin RL, Prato AV (1977) Radiological analysis of the mediastinum utilizing computed tomography. Radiol Clin North Am 15:309–329
32. Heitzman ER, Proto AV, Goldwin RL (1979) The role of computerized tomography in the diagnosis of diseases of the thorax. JAMA 241:933–936
33. Hessel SJ, Adams DF, Judy PF, Fishbein MC, Abrams HL (1978) Detection of myocardial ischemia in vitro by computed tomography. Radiology 127:413–418
34. Huang HK, Mazziotta JC (1978) Heart imaging from computerized tomography. Comput Tomogr 2:37–44
35. Husband JE, Fry KI (1980) The clinical implications of computed tomography on the detection and diagnosis of mediastinal disease. Br J Radiol 53:388
36. Hyson EA (1980) C.T. of esophagus. Incorrect labeling. AJR 135:425
37. Jansen W, Heuser L, Hombach V, Niehues B, Tauchert M, Behrenbe DW, Friedmann G, Hilger HH (1981) Der Einsatz nichtinvasiver Untersuchungsverfahren (Echokardiographie, Computertomographie) in der kardiologischen Notfalldiagnostik auf der Intensivstation. Intensivmed 18:310–318
38. Janson R, Lackner K, Grube E, Brecht G, Thurn P (1979) Computerkardiotomographie der idiopathischen hypertrophen subvalvulären Aortenstenose (IHSS)—ein neuartiger Beitrag zur nicht-invasiven Diagnose. Fortschr Röntgenstr 130(5):536–542
39. Kormano MJ, Dean PB, Hamlin DJ (1980) Upper extremity contrast medium infusion in computed tomography of upper mediastinal masses. J Comput Assist Tomogr 4:617–620
40. Köster O, Lackner K, Grube E, Thurn P (1981) Computertomographische Diagnostik kardialer, perikardialer und parakardialer Raumforderungen. Z Kardiol 70:733–741
41. Kreel L (1978) E.M.I. whole body scanner in long imaging. Br J Radiol 51:143–146
42. Kreel L (1979) Computed tomography of the thorax. Br J Radiol 52:83
43. Lackner K, Thurn P (1981) Computed tomography of the heart: ECG-gated and continuous scans. Radiol 140:413–420
44. Lackner K, Heuser L, Friedmann G, Thurn P (1978) Computerkardiotomographie bei Tumoren des kardialen Vorhofes. Fortschr Röntgenstr 129(6):735–739
45. Lackner K, Felix R, Oeser H, Wegener OH, Bücheler E, Buurman R, Heuser L, Mödder U (1979) Erweiterung der Röntgendiagnostik im Thoraxbereich durch die Computer-Tomographie. Radiologe 19:79–89
46. Lackner K, Thurn P, Orellano L, Schuppan U, Simon H, Kirchhof PG (1980) Der aortokoronare Bypass im Computertomogramm. Rofo 133(5):439–465

47. Lardé D, Belloir C, Vasile N, Frija J, Ferrané J (1980) Computed tomography of aortic dissection. Radiology 136:147–151

48. Lipton MJ, Hayashi TT, Boyd D, Carlsson E (1978) Measurement of left ventricular cast volume by computed tomography. Radiology 127:419–423

49. Lipton MJ, Carlsson E (1979) The diagnosis of ischemic heart disease by computed tomography. Ischemic Heart Dis 235–243

50. Long JA Jr, Doppman JL, Nienhuis AW (1980) Computed tomographic studies of thoracic extrame dullary hematopoiesis. J Comput Assist Tomogr 4:67–70

51. McLoud TC, Wittenberg J, Ferrucci JF Jr (1979) Computed tomography of the thorax and standard radiographic evaluation of the chest: a comparative study. J Comput Assist Tomogr 3:170–174

52. Mendez G, Isikoff MB, Isikoff SK, Sinner WN (1979) Fatty tumors of the thorax demonstrated by C.T. AJR 133:207–212

53. Mink JH, Bein ME, Sukov R, Herrman C, Winter J, Sample WF, Mulder D (1978) Computed tomography of anterior mediastinum in patients with myasthenia gravis suspected thymoma. AJR 130:239–246

54. Modic MT, Janicki PC (1980) Computed tomography of mass lesions of the right cardiophrenic angle. J Comput Assist Tomogr 4:521–526

55. Moncada R, Salinas M, Churchill R, Love L, Reynes C, Demos TC, Hale D, Schreiber R (1980) Patency of saphenous aortocoronary-bypass grafts demonstrated by computed tomography. Neth J Med 303(9):503–505

56. Mountain CF, Carr DT, Anderson WAD (1974) Clinical staging of lung cancer. AJR 120:130–138

57. Nair CK, Sketch MH, Mahoney PD, Lynch JD, Mooss AN, Kenn NP (1981) Detection of left ventricular thrombi by computerised tomography. Br Heart J 45:535–541

58. Onitsuka H, Kuhns LR (1980) Dextro convexity of the mediastinum in the azygoesophageal recess: a normal C.T. variant in young adults. Radiology 135:126

59. Osteaux M, Jeanmart L, Struyven J, Huvenne R (1978) Head and trunk. Springer, Berlin Heidelberg New York, pp 162–168

60. Owens GR, Arger PH, Mulhern CB Jr, Coleman BG, Gohel V (1980) C.T. evaluation of mediastinal pseudocyst. J Comput Assist Tomogr 4:256–259

61. Powell WJ, Wittenberg J, Miller SW, Maturi RA, Dinsmore RE (1979) Assessment of drug intervention on the ischemic myocardium: serial imaging and measurement with computerized tomography. Am J Cardiol 44:46–52

62. Pugatch RD, Faling LJ, Robbins AH, Snider GL (1978) Differentiation of pleural and pulmonary lesions using computed tomography. J Comput Assist Tomogr 2:601–606

63. Pugatch RD, Faling LJ, Robbins AH, Spira R (1980) C.T. diagnosis of benign mediastinal abnormalities. AJR 134:685–694

64. Rohlfing BM, Korobkin M, Hall AD (1977) Computed tomography of intrathoracic omental herniation and other mediastinal fatty masses. J Comput Assist Tomogr 1:181–183

65. Roy-Camille R (1959) Coupes horizontales du tronc. Masson, Paris

66. Ritman EL, Robb RA, Johnson SA, Chevalier PA, Gilbert BK, Greenleaf JF, Sturm RE, Wood EH (1978) Quantitative imaging of the structure and function of the heart, lungs, and circulation. Mayo Clin Proc 53:3–11

67. Robb RA, Ritman EL (1979) High speed synchronous volume computed tomography of the heart. Radiology 133:655–661

68. Sagel SS, Weiss ES, Gillard RG, Hounsfield GN, Jost RGT, Stanley RJ, Ter-Pogossian MM (1977) Gated computed tomography of the human heart. Invest Radiol 12:563–566

69. Scanlan JG, Gustafson DE, Chevalier PA, Robb RA, Ritman EL (1980) Evaluation of ischemic heart disease with a prototype volume imaging computed tomographic (CT) scanner: preliminary experiments. Am J Cardiol 46:1263–1268

70. Schad N, Schepke P, Rohde U, Schepke H, Schmid V, Breit A (1981) Timing of exposure in angiographic computed tomography. Cardiovasc Intervent Radiol 4:59–65

71. Shevland JE, Chiu LC, Shapiro RL, Young JA, Rossi NP (1978) The role of conventional tomography and computed tomography in assessing the resectability of primary lung cancer: a preliminary report. CT 2:1–19

72. Siemers PT, Higgins CB, Schmidt W, Ashburn W, Hagan P (1978) Detection, quantitation and contrast enhancement of myocardial infarctions utilizing computerized axial tomography: comparison with histochemical staining and Tc-pyrophosphate imaging. Invest Radiol 13:103–109

73. Ter-Pogossian MM, Weiss ES, Coleman RE, Sobel BE (1976) Computed tomography of the heart. Am J Roentgenol 127:79–90

74. Tomoda H, Hoshiai M, Furuya H, Shotsu A, Ootaki M, Matsuyama S (1981) Evaluation of left ventricular thrombus with computed tomography. Am J Cardiol 48:573–577

75. Underwood GH Jr, Hooper RG, Axelbaum SP, Goodwin DW (1979) C.T. scanning of the thorax in the staging of bronchogenic carcinoma. N Engl J Med 300:777–778

76. Vasile N, Usdin JP, Belloir C, Ferrane J, Galey JJ, Vernant P (1979) Perméabilité des pontages aorto-coronaries explorés par tomodensitométric. Arch. Mal. Cœur 11:1346–1351

77. Wittenberg J, Powell J, Dinsmore RE, Miller SW, Maturi RA (1977) Computerized tomography of ischemic myocardium: quantitation of exten and severity of edema in an in vitro canine model. Invest Radiol 12:215–223

CHAPTER 5

Spine

D. Baleriaux, L. Divano, N. Hermanus, M. Lemort,
M. Stienon, and L. Ticket

5.1 Introduction

This chapter illustrates and summarizes 5 years experience of spinal CT, which has gained increasing importance in the radiological assessment of spinal disease. Its technical performance is constantly and rapidly improving, enabling more and more accurate study of the spinal structures, which are visualized very well with the axial approach. Reconstruction programs in different spatial planes provide interesting complementary information, and the specific densitometric approach often permits a precise etiological diagnosis.

The difficulty of localizing the studied level is nowadays overcome by the use of digital radiographic devices incorporated into the scanner (e.g. toposcan, scout view). This "computer radiograph" can also be used to calculate the gantry inclination needed to obtain precise axial sections of the spine. The use of thin (2-mm) slices allows the evaluation of very small anatomical structures by lessening the partial volume effect.

Computer tomography of the spine can be performed in different ways:

1. Examination without any preparation: "native" CT. This is most valuable in the assessment of bony structures and is growing in application with increasing spatial and densitometric resolution.

2. Examination after intravenous injection of contrast medium. The epidural space is more clearly defined and the medulla can more often be evaluated. Vascular and highly vascularized structures are visualized. This method is used for the first study of spinal canal content and in seeking highly vascularized tumours such as meningiomas and neurinomas.

3. Examination after intrathecal injection of water-soluble contrast medium, as a complement to conventional myelography or as a primary examination. In the latter case, the concentration of the contrast medium used can be decreased. This "computed myelography" is specially indicated in the search for intraspinal processes. It allows accurate demarcation of the medulla and the nerve roots. In contrast to conventional myelography, a complete arrest of the progress of contrast medium by intraspinal processes is observed only exceptionally with CT because of the high densitometric resolution. CT thus easily affords a more precise evaluation of the extent of these lesions.

In summary, CT offers a global morphological approach to the spine and enables better physiological study of the spinal cord and nerve roots seen within soft and bony envelopes.

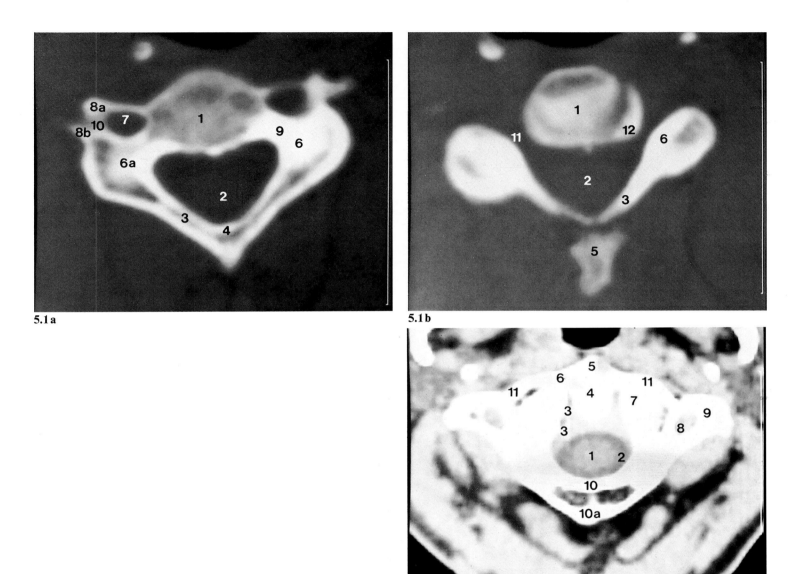

5.1a

5.1b

5.2

Fig. 5.1a, b. Normal aspect of a cervical vertebra. **a** "Pedicular" level; **b** "discal" level.

1 Vertebral body
2 Vertebral foramen
3 Lamina
4 Posterior arch
5 Spinal process
6 Transverse process with superior articular facet (*6a*)
7 Transverse foramen
8 Anterior (*a*) and posterior (*b*) tubercles
9 Pedicle
10 Sulcus for spinal nerve
11 Intervertebral foramen
12 Unciform process

Fig. 5.2. Normal C1–C2 native scan.

1 Medulla (clearly defined at this level)
2 Subarachnoid space
3 Epidural space
4 Odontoid process of the axis
5 Anterior tubercle
6 Anterior arch of C1
7 Superior articular facet
8 Transverse foramen
9 Transverse process
10 Posterior arch of C1 with posterior tubercle (*10a*)
11 Lateral mass

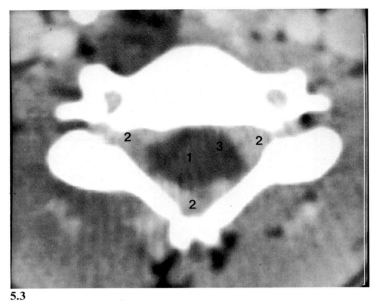

5.3

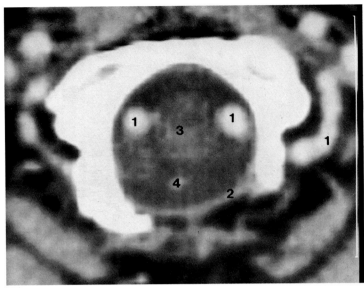

5.4

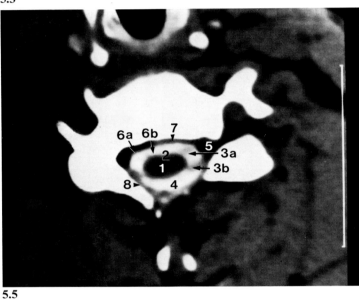

5.5

Fig. 5.3. Normal cervical vertebra after intravenous contrast injection. The epidural space is enhanced

1 Medulla
2 Enhanced epidural tissue
3 Intradural space

Fig. 5.4. Normal aspect of the foramen magnum after intravenous contrast injection.

1 Vertebral arteries
2 Enhancement of envelopes
3 Medulla oblongata (well visualized at this level)
4 Posterior inferior cerebellar artery

Fig. 5.5. Typical cervical computed myelography at lower levels (C3–C7).

1 Oval medullar outline
2 Anterior sulcus
3 Anterior (*a*) and posterior (*b*) nerve roots
4 Enhanced subarachnoid space
5 Epidural space
6 Meningeal layers: dura mater, arachnoid (*6a*) and pia mater (*6b*)
7 Longitudinal posterior ligament
8 Ligamentum flavum

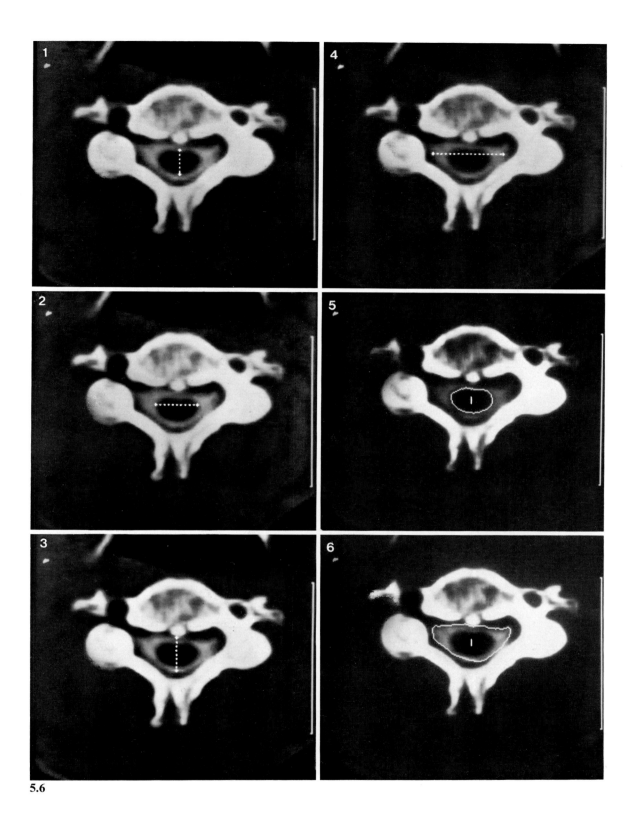

5.6

Fig. 5.6. Computed myelography study of the normal values of medullar diameters. Measurements were made with standard settings of centre (200 HU) and window width (600 HU).

1 Anteroposterior medullar diameter
2 Transverse medullar diameter
3 Anteroposterior diameter of the dural sac

4 Transverse diameter of the dural sac
5 Medullar area
6 Dural area

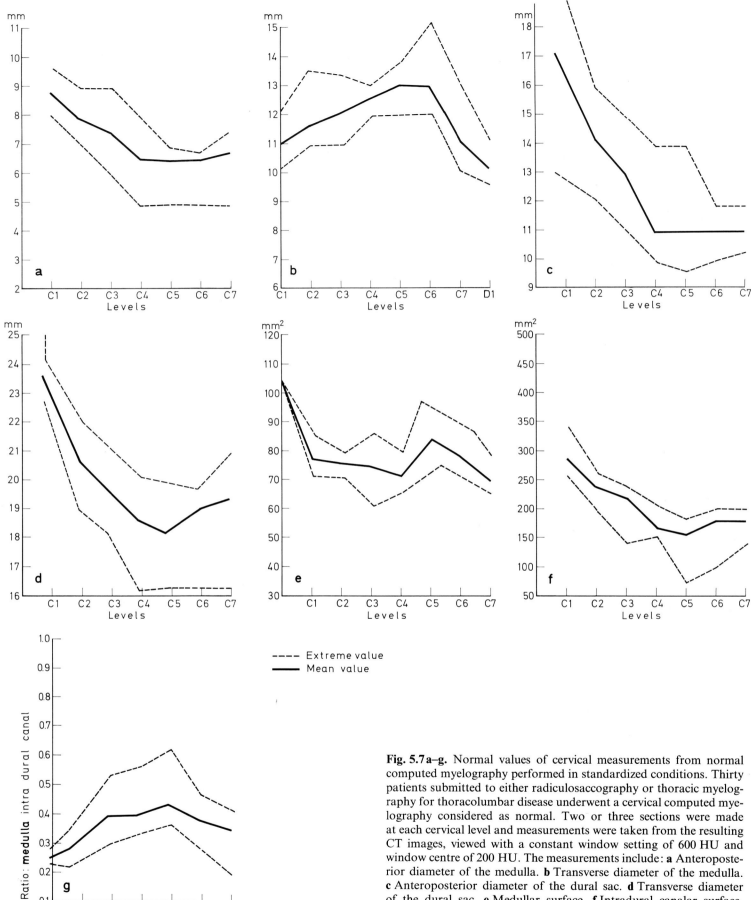

Fig. 5.7a–g. Normal values of cervical measurements from normal computed myelography performed in standardized conditions. Thirty patients submitted to either radiculosaccography or thoracic myelography for thoracolumbar disease underwent a cervical computed myelography considered as normal. Two or three sections were made at each cervical level and measurements were taken from the resulting CT images, viewed with a constant window setting of 600 HU and window centre of 200 HU. The measurements include: **a** Anteroposterior diameter of the medulla. **b** Transverse diameter of the medulla. **c** Anteroposterior diameter of the dural sac. **d** Transverse diameter of the dural sac. **e** Medullar surface. **f** Intradural canalar surface. **g** Ratio of medullar surface to intradural surface

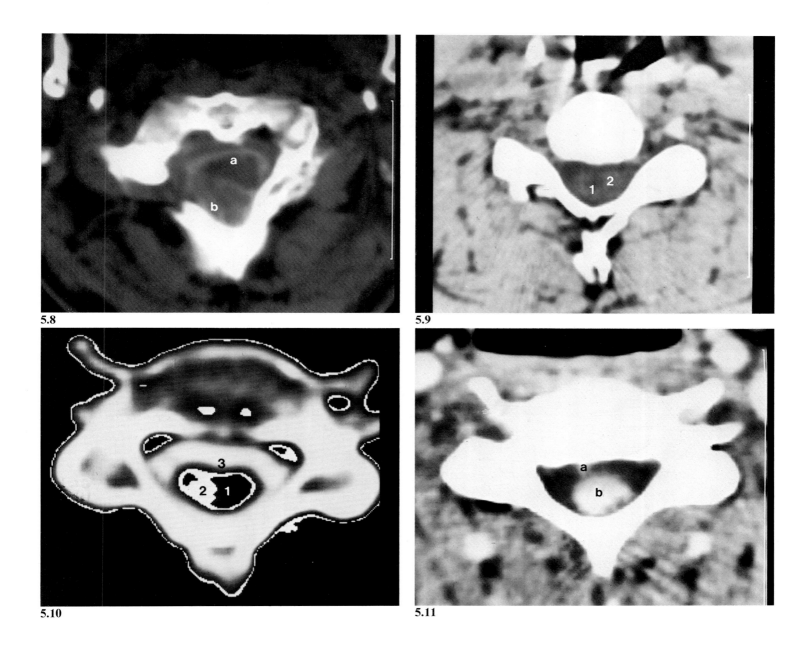

5.8

5.9

5.10

5.11

Fig. 5.8. Malformation of the craniovertebral region: basilar impression. Computed myelography at C2 level shows cerebellar herniation. Note the very abnormally shaped medulla (*a*) and the tonsil of the cerebellum (*b*)

Fig. 5.10. Syringomyelia. On computed myelography, "highlighting" emphasizes the hyperdense intramedullar cavity.

1 Medulla
2 Intramedullar syringomyelic pouch filled with metrizamide
3 Enhanced subarachnoid space (metrizamide)

Fig. 5.9. Syringomyelia. A native scan clearly demonstrates a hypodense round area (*1*) within the spinal cord (*2*)

Fig. 5.11. Medullar haemangioblastoma in von Hippel-Lindau disease. A CT scan with intravenous contrast injection shows tortuous vessels (*a*) associated with the highly vascularized tumour and tumoral malformation (*b*)

127

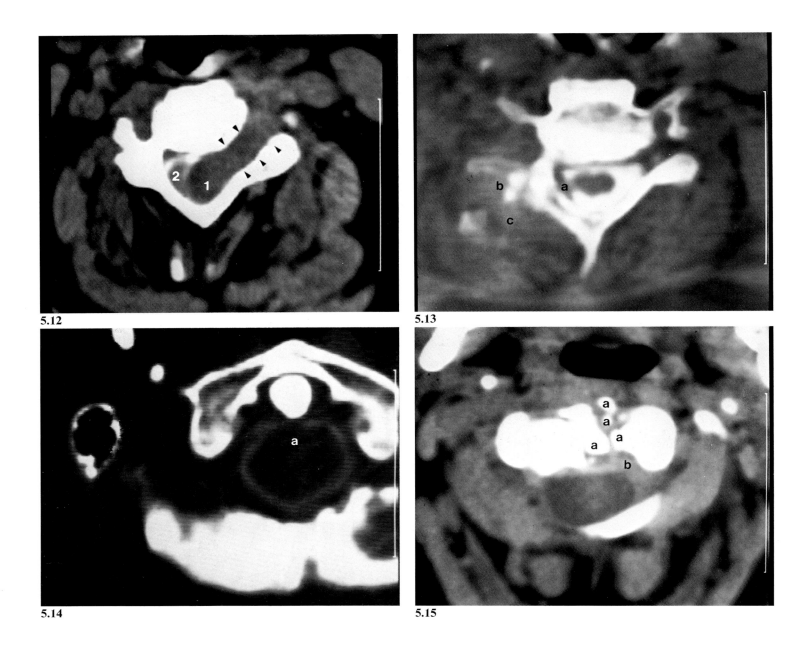

5.12

5.13

5.14

5.15

Fig. 5.13. Carcinomatous epiduritis. Computed myelography reveals infiltrated epidural tissue (*a*), partial destruction of the left transverse process (*b*) and tumoral infiltration into the paravertebral soft tissues (*c*).

CT differentiates between epidural tumoral extension from canalar stenosis caused by metastatic vertebral collapse

Fig. 5.12. Cervical neurinoma. Computed myelography shows a large neurinoma (*1*) displacing the medulla (*2*) and enlarging the intervertebral foramen (*arrowheads*)

Fig. 5.14. Cervical glioblastoma at the C1–C2 level and craniovertebral region. Computer myelography shows significant enlargement of the spinal cord (*a*)

Fig. 5.15. Fracture of the base of the odontoïd process of C2. There are multiple bony fragments (*a*). Note the enlargement of the epidural space (*b*) adjacent to the fracture site

128

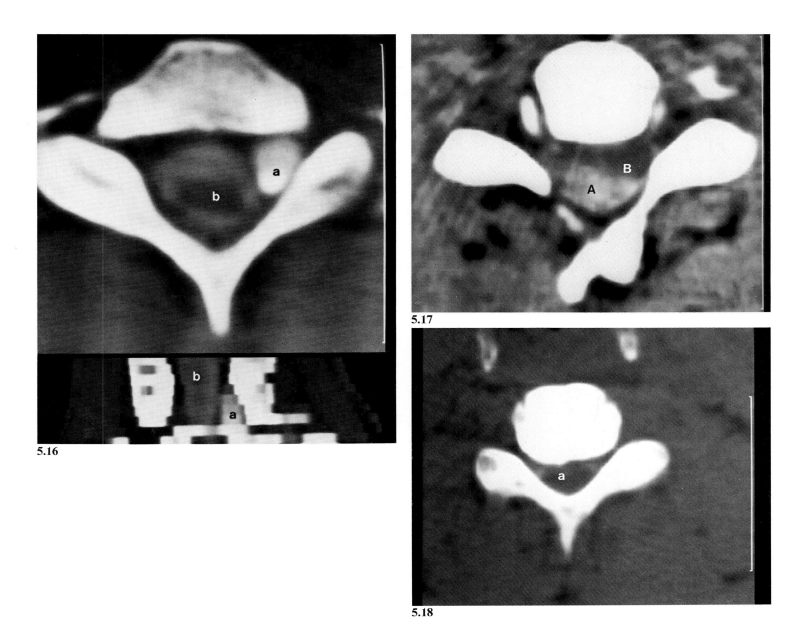

5.16

5.17

5.18

Fig. 5.16. Traumatic rupture of the brachial plexus. Computed myelography with frontal reconstruction shows filling of a pseudocyst with contrast medium (*a*). The cervical nerve root is not seen on this side. There is contralateral displacement of the medulla (*b*)

Fig. 5.17. Spontaneous epidural haemorrhage during delivery. A native cervical scan shows a fresh epidural haematoma (*A*) (spontaneously hyperdense area) and medullar displacement (*B*)

Fig. 5.18. Cervical stenosis. Computed myelography shows reduced canalar lumen with compression of the spinal cord (*a*)

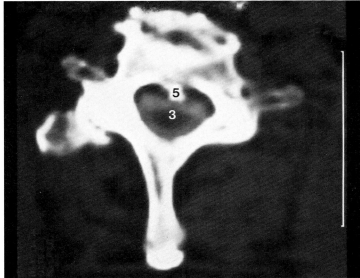

5.19a

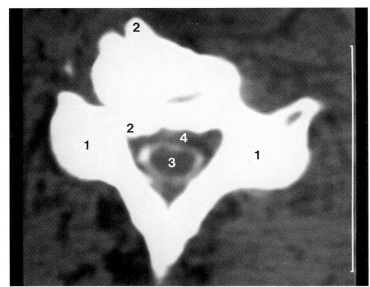

5.19b

Fig. 5.19a, b. Cervical arthrosic myelopathy. **a, b** Computed myelography at pedicular level reveals posterior marginal osteophytosis. There is hypertrophy of the articular processes (*1*), huge bony marginal apposition (*2*), slight posterior displacement of the medulla (*3*) and enlargement of the epidural space by ligamentous hypertrophy (*4*). A hard hernia (*5*) may displace the medulla even further posteriorly

Fig. 5.20. Huge medial soft disc herniation. CT scan with intravenous contrast injection at pedicular level shows that the anteroposterior canalar diameter is much reduced! The central hypodense zone (*1*) corresponds to the true discal hernia, while the arciform contrast enhancement (*2*) points to the displaced longitudinal ligament and meningeal layers

Fig. 5.21a, b. Soft discs herniation at C6–C7 level. **a** Native scan; **b** computed myelography. These two cases of anterolateral disc herniation exhibit reduced subarachnoïd space, left nerve root compression and slightly displaced medulla.

1 Herniated disc   *2* Spinal cord

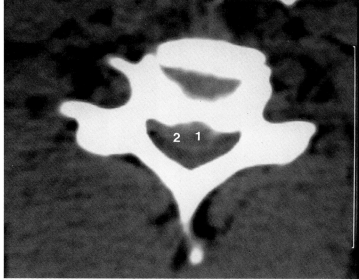

5.20

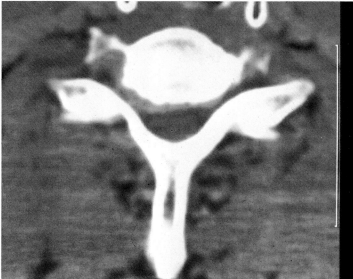

5.21a

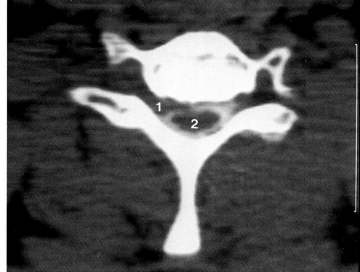

5.21b

130

5.4 Thoracic Spine: Normal Anatomy

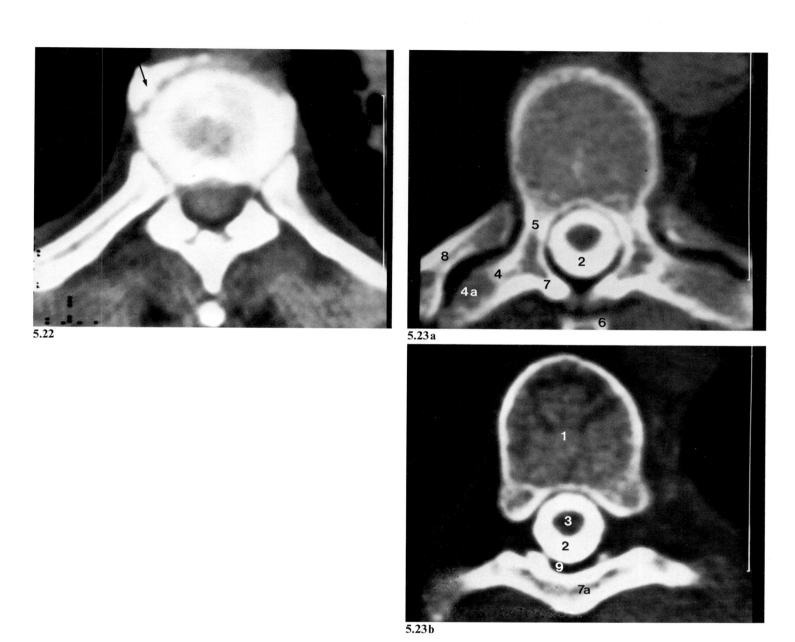

5.22

5.23a

5.23b

Fig. 5.22. Anterior marginal osteophytosis. A native thoracic CT scan at discal level reveals the osteophytosis (*arrow*).

The thoracic spinal cord is not seen satisfactorily on a plain CT scan

Fig. 5.23a, b. Normal thoracic computed myelography. **a** Pedicular level; **b** Foraminal level.

1 Vertebral body
2 Subarachnoïd space
3 Spinal cord (rounded shape)
4 Transverse process with costal articulation process (*4a*)
5 Pedicle
6 Spinal process
7 Lamina
7a Lamina of overlying vertebra
8 Rib
9 Epidural space

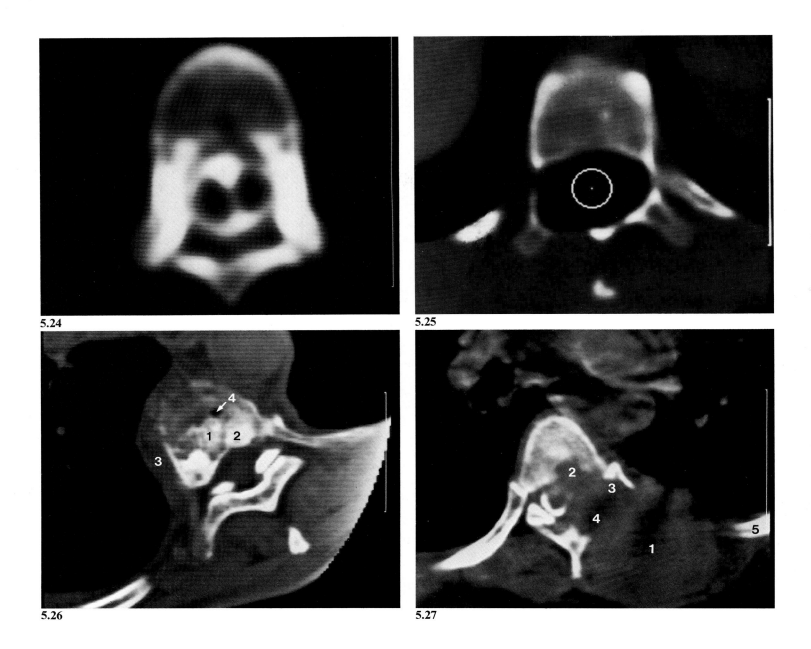

5.24

5.25

5.26

5.27

Fig. 5.24. Diastematomyelia demonstrated by computed myelography (Courtesy Dr. C. Marsault, Department of Radiology (Head: Prof. J. Ferrané, Hospital H. Mondor, Créteil, France

Fig. 5.26. Thoracic spondylodiscitis. Native CT scan shows bony changes (*1*) with protrusion of bone fragments into the spinal canal (*2*), and displaced paraspinal lines (*3*). The presence of small gaseous images (*4*) points to an infectious origin. Courtesy Dr. D. Lardé, Department of Radiology (Head: Prof. J. Ferrané, Hospital H. Mondor, Créteil, France)

Fig. 5.25. Thoracic epidural cyst. Enlargement of the thoracic spinal canal with bony sclerosis is evident. The intracanalar values indicate purely homogeneous water-like densities

Fig. 5.27. Pott's disease: tuberculous abscess at the thoracic level. Computed myelography reveals a huge heterogeneous soft tissue lesion (*1*) destroying the partly adjacent bony structures: posterior part of vertebral body (*2*), pedicle (*3*), posterior arch (*4*), rib (*5*). There is tumour-like infiltration of the thoracic spinal canal, with epiduritis and spinal cord compression

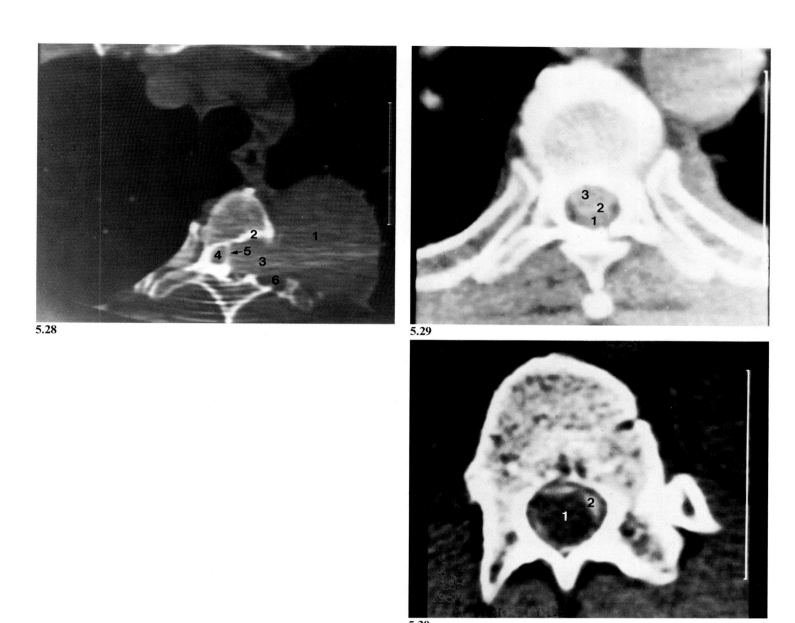

5.28

5.29

5.30

Fig. 5.28. Thoracic neurinoma. Several signs are revealed on computed myelography. Courtesy Dr. D. Lardé and Dr. C. Marsault, Department of Diagnostic Radiology (Head: Prof. J. Ferrané, Hospital H. Mondor, Créteil, France)

1 Large benign tumoral mass extending into the left posterior costo-vertebral gutter
2 Osseous erosion of the vertebral body: sharp limits with peripheral osteosclerosis
3 Considerable enlargement of the intervertebral foramen
4 Displacement of the spinal cord
5 Compression, but not infiltration of the dural sac
6 Bony erosion of the lamina, transverse process and rib

Fig. 5.29. Thoracic epidural carcinomatosis. Computed myelography reveals irregular tumoral thickening of the posterior epidural tissues (*1*) impinging on the subarachnoïd space (*2*) and causing forward displacement of the spinal cord (*3*). There is no tumoral infiltration of bone

Fig. 5.30. Thoracic intramedullar metastasis of an intraventricular meningiosarcoma. Computed myelography shows progressive enlargement of the spinal cord (*1*), which presents irregular borders. Correspondingly, the subarachnoïd space (*2*) is progressively reduced

133

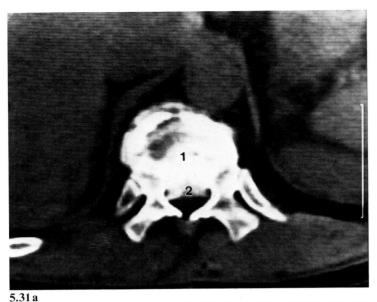

5.31 a

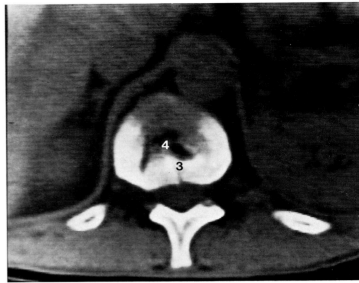

5.31 b

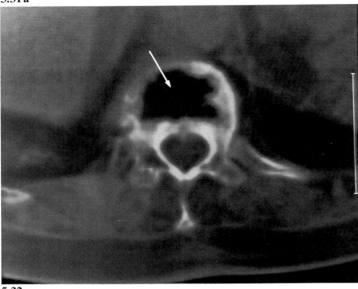

5.32

Fig. 5.31a, b. Traumatic lesions of bone and disc. **a** A native scan at T12 pedicular level shows a fracture of the vertebral body (*1*), with displacement of the posterior wall (*2*) reducing canalar diameters. **b** A native scan at the T12–L1 discal level reveals a fracture of the vertebral plate (*3*) and a vacuum disc phenomenon (*4*) probably related to discal traction. Courtesy Dr. D. Lardé, Department of Radiology (Head: Prof. J. Ferrané, Hospital H. Mondor, Créteil, France)

Fig. 5.32. Vacuum phenomenon of the vertebral body: Maldague's syndrome. A thoracic native scan shows ischaemic collapse of the spongiosa with intact vertebral cortex. There is no reaction of the paravertebral tissues, in contrast to infectious lesions. Courtesy Dr. D. Lardé, Department of Radiology (Head: Prof. J. Ferrané, Hospital H. Mondor, Créteil, France)

134

5.6 Lumbosacral Spine: Normal Anatomy and Computed Myelography

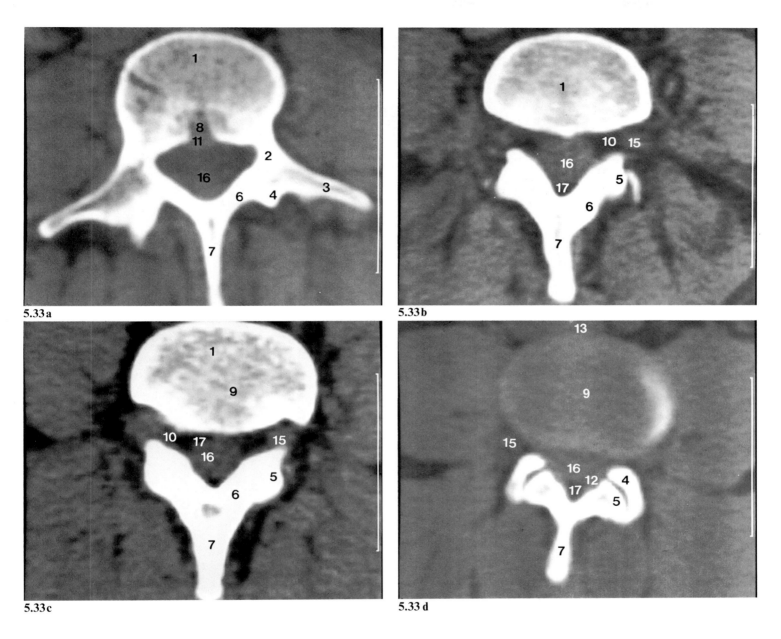

5.33 a

5.33 b

5.33 c

5.33 d

Fig. 5.33 a–d. Normal native CT scan at lumbar level. **a** Pedicular section; **b, c** subpedicular section; **d** discal section.

1 Vertebral body
2 Vertebral pedicle
3 Transverse process
4 Superior articular process
5 Inferior articular process
6 Lamina
7 Spinous process
8 Basivertebral veins
9 Intervertebral disc
10 Intervertebral foramen
11 Posterior longitudinal ligament
12 Ligamentum flavum

13 Anterior longitudinal ligament
14 Spinal nerves
15 Spinal ganglions
16 Dural sac
17 Epidural space
18 Epidural veins
19 Conus medullaris
20 Cauda equina
22 Abdominal aorta
23 Crura
24 Psoas muscle
25 Sacrospinalis muscle

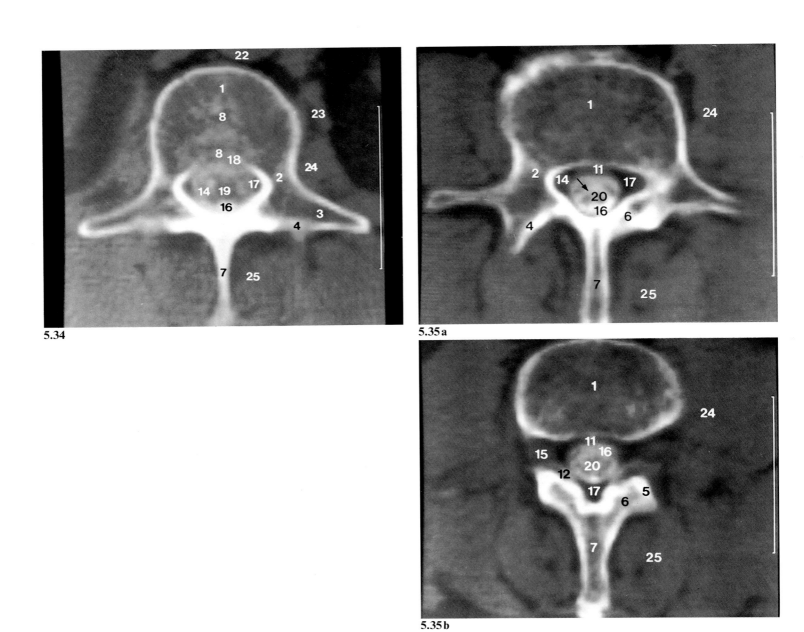

Fig. 5.34. Normal computed myelosaccography at L1. Pedicular level. Note the typical X-shaped aspect of the conus medullaris.

For key to numbers see Fig. 5.33 legend

Fig. 5.35a, b. Normal computed radiculosaccography at L4 level. **a** Pedicular section; **b** lower subpedicular section.

For key to numbers see Fig. 5.33 legend

136

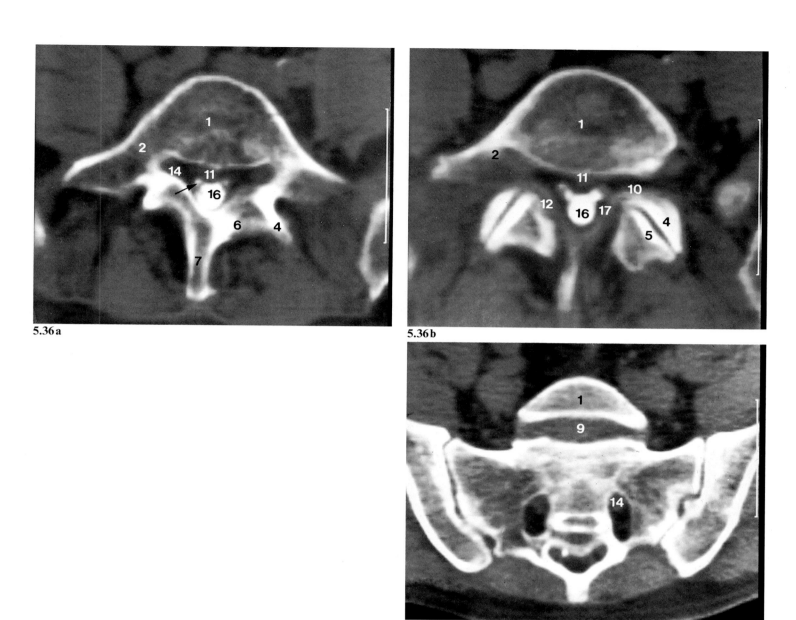

5.36 a

5.36 b

5.37

Fig. 5.36 a, b. Normal computed radiculosaccography at L5. **a** Typical pedicular section; **b** subpedicular section.

For key to numbers see Fig. 5.33 legend

Fig. 5.37. Normal native CT scan of the sacrum. Note the good visibility of the sacral nerve roots.

For key to numbers see Fig. 5.33 legend

137

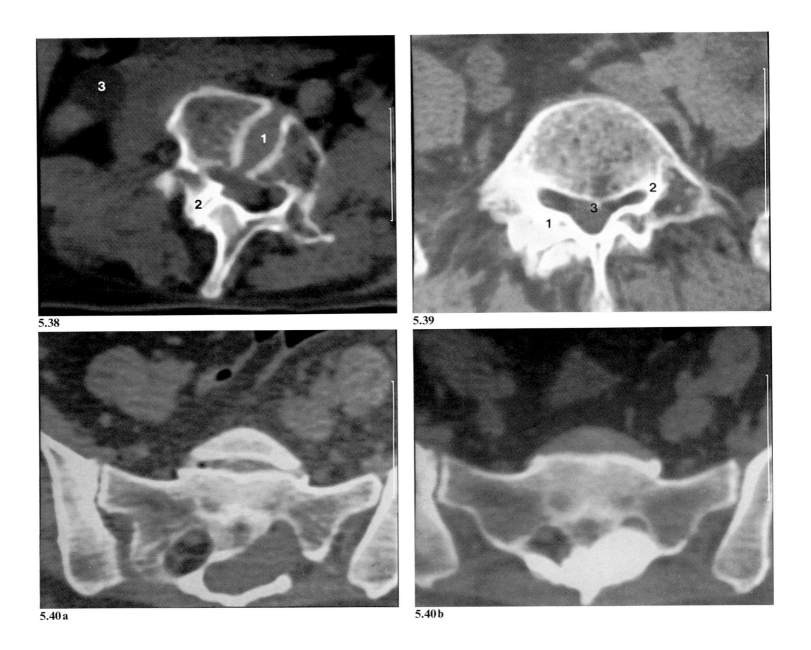

5.38

5.39

5.40a

5.40b

Fig. 5.38. Congenital somatoschisis. A native scan shows butterfly vertebra. There is significant cyphoscoliosis and the canal is narrow.

1 Sagittal vertebral cleft
2 Unilateral spondylolysis
3 Renal cyst

Fig. 5.40a, b. Extradural arachnoïd cyst. **a** Native CT scan of the sacrum; **b** computer radiculosaccography. A large cystic cavity is causing bony lesions

Fig. 5.39. Congenital narrow lumbar canal. A native scan at pedicular level reveals a decrease in anteroposterior canalar diameter, heart-shaped lumen, hypertrophy of the articular facets (*1*) and shortness of the vertebral pedicles (*2*). Note the normal little osseous cap in front of the penetration point of the basivertebral veins (*3*)

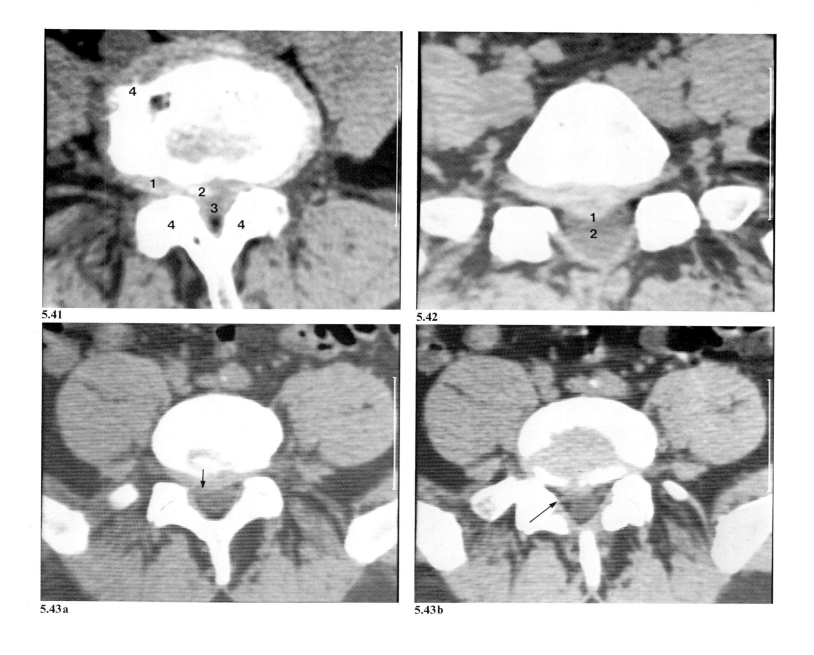

5.41

5.42

5.43 a

5.43 b

Fig. 5.41. Narrow lumbar canal with L4–L5 discal herniation. A native scan shows several significant features.

1 Discal herniation
2 Partly calcified disc
3 Dural sac with reduced lumen
4 Arthrosic degenerative lesions

Fig. 5.42. Soft, medial L5–S1 discal herniation. A native scan shows the herniation (*1*) and the dural sac (*2*)

Fig. 5.43a, b. Left posterior L5–S1 disc herniation. There is a soft tissue density mass, with posterior displacement of the left S1 root, absence of epidural fat and encroachment upon the dural sac (*arrows*)

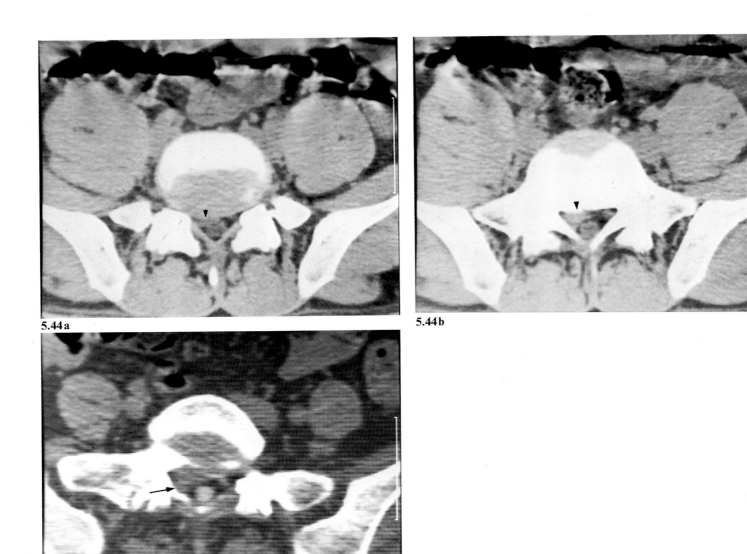

5.44 a

5.44 b

5.45

Fig. 5.44a, b. L5–S1 disc herniation. Note the soft tissue mass arising from the L5–S1 disc (*arrowheads*) behind the body of S1, with marked displacement of the S1 root

Fig. 5.45. L5–S1 disc herniation. There is lateralization of the hernia to the left, with displacement of the left S1 root (*arrow*). Note also the absence of epidural fat

140

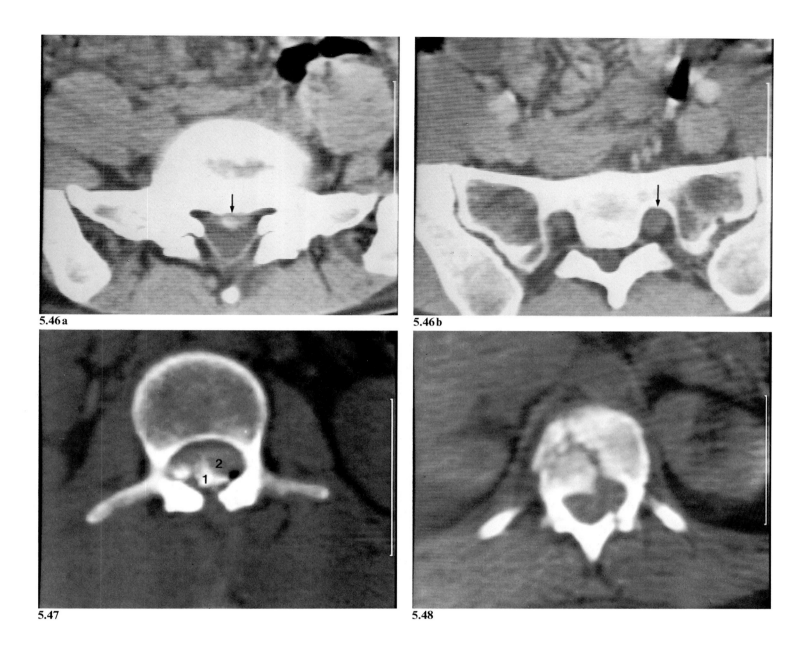

5.46a

5.46b

5.47

5.48

Fig. 5.46a, b. Calcified disc herniation. **a** A plain scan at the level of S1, a few millimetres below L5–S1, shows a medial disc herniation with a calcified posterior border (*arrow*). **b** A section through the S1 roots reveals increased diameter of the right root (*arrow*). This is rarely seen and is thought to represent oedema of the root

Fig. 5.47. Postoperative lumbar arachnoïditis. Computed radiculosac-cography shows the subarachnoïd space (*1*) and agglutinated nerve roots (*2*)

Fig. 5.48. Fracture of T12 and L1. The canalar lumen displays a reduced cross-sectional area

141

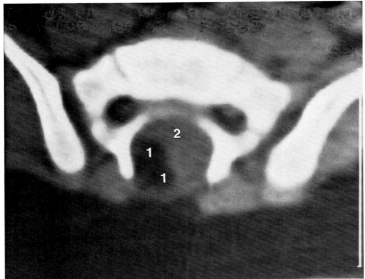

Fig. 5.49. Sacral lipoma in a child. A native CT scan at sacral level shows a lipoma presenting typical fatty densities (*1*) and the dural sac (*2*). There is associated enlargement of the lumbosacral canal

5.49

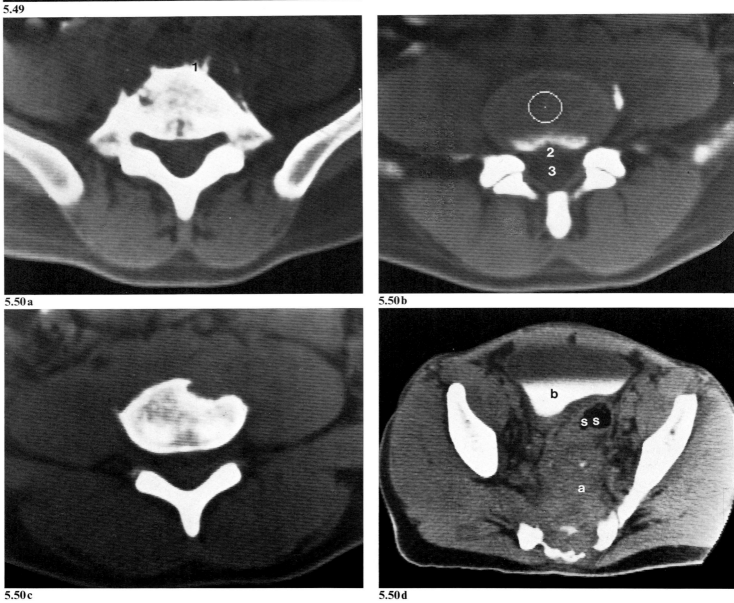

5.50a

5.50b

5.50c

5.50d

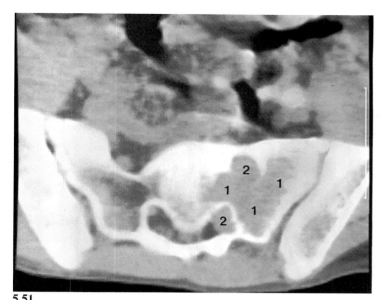

5.51

Fig. 5.51. Ewing sarcoma of the rib with sacral metastasis.

1 Tumoral infiltration of bony structures
2 Tumoral filling of right sacral foramina

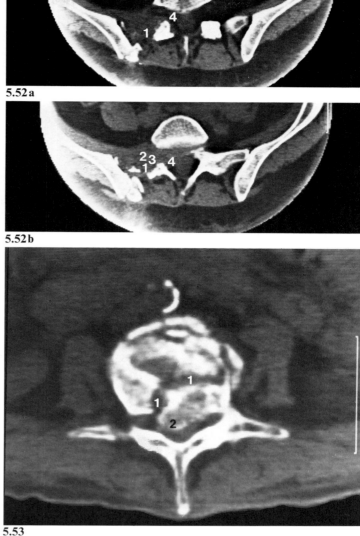

5.52a

5.52b

5.53

◁ **Fig. 5.50a–d.** Tuberculous L4–L5 spondylodiscitis with presacral and sacral tuberculous abscess. **a** Discrete osteolytic lesions of anterior part of body of L5, with spicular formations due to periostal reaction (*17*). **b** The L4–L5 intervertebral disc has a mean density value of 69.5 HU. Evident are the normal epidural space (*2*) and the dural sac (*3*). **c** A CT scan at L4 level reveals a sharply defined osteolytic lesion of the anterior part of vertebral body, with slight periostal reaction. **d** Large osteolytic lesion of the anterior sacrum. A huge presacral abscess (*a*) forces back the sigmoïd (*s*) and the bladder (*b*). Courtesy Dr. D. Lardé, Department of Radiology (Head: Prof. J. Ferrané, Hospital H. Mondor, Créteil, France)

Fig. 5.52a, b. Primary malignant osseous tumour of the left sacral wing. Courtesy Dr. D. Lardé, Department of Radiology (Head: Prof. J. Ferrané, Hospital H. Mondor, Créteil, France)

1 Tumoral mass infiltration
2 Presacral soft tissue
3 Articular process
4 Extension into the spinal canal: enlarged anterior and left lateral epidural space

Fig. 5.53. Neoplastic infiltration of L3 by lung metastasis. A native CT scan shows a pathological fracture of the vertebral body (*1*) and backward displacement of the posterior wall of the vertebral body (*2*) into the vertebral foramen with compression of radicular elements. CT allows the differential diagnosis between secondary compression of radicular elements by protrusion of bony fragments and that by epiduritis. Courtesy Dr. Lardé, Department of Radiology (Head: Prof. J. Ferrané, Hospital H. Mondor, Créteil, France)

143

References

1. Balériaux-Waha D, Mortelmans LL, Dupont MG, Jeanmart L (1977) Computed tomography for lesions of the craniovertebral region. Neuroradiology 13:59–61
2. Balériaux-Waha D, Osteaux M, Terwinghe G, de Meeus A, Jeanmart L (1977) The management of anterior sacral meningocele with computed tomography. Neuroradiology 14:45–46
3. Balériaux-Waha D, Rétif J, Noterman J, Terwinghe G, Mortelmans LL, Dupont MG, Jeanmart L (1978) C.t. scanning for the diagnosis of the cerebellar and spinal lesions of von Hippel-Lindau's disease. Neuroradiology 14:241–244
4. Balériaux-Waha D, Terwinghe G, Jeanmart L (1977) The value of computed tomography for the diagnosis of hourglass tumors of the spine. Neuroradiology 14:31–32
5. Balériaux-Waha D, Sœur M, Stadnik T, Lemaitre Y, Jeanmart L (1980) C.T. of the adult spine with metrizamide. In: Post JD (ed) Radiographic evaluation of the spine. Masson, New York, p 353–365
6. Bonafé A, Ethier R, Melançon D, Belanger G, Peters T (1980) High-resolution computed tomography in cervical syringomyelia. J Comput Assist Tomogr 4:42–47
7. Carrera GF, Haughton VM, Syvertsen A, Williams AM (1980) C.T. of lumbar facet joints. Radiology 134:145–148
8. Colley D, Dunsker S (1978) Traumatic narrowing of the dorsolumbar spinal canal demonstrated by computed tomography. Radiology 129:95–98
9. Di Chiro G, Axelbaum Sp, Schellinger D, Twigg H, Ledley R (1976) Computerized axial tomography in syringomyelia. N Engl J Med 292:13–16
10. Di Chiro G, Schellinger D (1976) Computed tomography of spinal cord after lumbar intrathecal introduction of metrizamide (computer assisted myelography). Radiology 120:101–104
11. Fauber EN, Wolpert SM, Scott RM, Belking SC, Carter BL (1979) C.T. of spinal fracture. J Comput Assist Tomogr 3:657–661
12. Federle MP, Moss AA, Margolin FR (1980) Role of computed tomography in patients with "sciatica". J Comput Assist Tomogr 4:335–341
13. Hammerschlag S, Wolpert S, Carter B (1976) Computed tomography of the spinal canal. Radiology 121:361–367
14. Haughton V, Syvertsen A, Williams A (1980) Soft tissue anatomy within the spinal canal as seen on computed tomography. Radiology 134:649–655
15. James HE, Oliff M (1977) Computed tomography in spinal dysraphism. J Comput Assist Tomogr 1:391–397
16. Kramer L, Krouth G (1978) Computerized tomography. An adjacent to early diagnosis in the cauda equina syndrome of ankylosing spondylitis. Arch Neurol 35:116–118
17. Kreel L, Osborn S (1976) Transverse axial tomography of the spinal column: a comparison of anatomical specimens with EMI scan appearences. Radiology 42:73–80
18. Krol G, Khomeini R, Deck MF (1978) C.T. of the spine. Neuroradiology 16:362–363
19. Lee B, Kazam E, Newman A (1978) Computed tomography of the spine and spinal cord. Radiology 128:95–102
20. Maldague B, Noel H, Malghem J (1978) The Intravertebral vacuum cleft: a sign of ischemic vertebral collapse. Radiology 129:23–29
21. Meyer G, Haughton V, Williams A (1979) Diagnosis of herniated lumbar disk with computed tomography. N Engl J Med 301:1166
22. Nagawaka H, Juang VP, Malis LI, Wolf BS (1977) C.T. of intraspinal and paraspinal neoplasm. J Comput Assist Tomogr 1:377–390
23. Nardick T, King D, Moran C, Sagel S (1980) Computed tomography of the lumbar thecal sac. J Comput Assist Tomogr 4:37–41
24. Oberson R, Azam F (1978) C.A.T. of the spine and spinal cord. Neuroradiology 16:369–370
25. Oberson R, Azam F, Dufresne JJ, Pagani JP, Perrig A, Regli F, Zdrojewski B (1978) Tomographie axiale computérisée de la mœlle et du canal rachidien. Med Hyg 36:2489–2496
26. Resjö M, Harwood-Nash D, Fitz C, Chuang S (1979) Computed tomographic metrizamide myelography in syringohydromyelia. Radiology 131:405–407
27. Resjö M, Harwood-Nash D, Fitz C, Chuang S (1979) Normal cord in infants and children examined with computed tomographic metrizamide myelography. Radiology 130:691–696
28. Roub L, Drager B (1979) Spinal computed tomography: limitations and applications. AJR 133:267–273
29. Scotti L (1977) Computed tomography of the spinal canal and cord. Comput Tomogr 1:229–234
30. Sheldon J, Sersland T, Leborgne J (1977) Computed tomography of the lower lumbar vertebral column. Normal anatomy and the stenotic canal. Radiology 124:113–118
31. Tadmor R, Davis K, Roberson G, New P, Taveras J (1978) Computed tomographic evaluation of traumatic spinal injuries. Radiology 127:825–827
32. Taylor A, Haughton V, Doust B (1980) C.T. imaging of the thoracic spinal cord without intrathecal contrast medium. J Comp Assist Tomogr 4(2):223–224
33. Thyssen U, Keyser A, Horstink M, Meyer I (1979) Morphology of the cervical spinal cord on computed myelography. Neuroradiology 18:57–62
34. Ulrich C, Binet E, Sanecki M, Kieffer S Quantitative assessment of the lumbar spinal canal by computed tomography.
35. Weinstein M, Rothner D, Duchesneau P, Dohn D (1975) Computed tomography in diastematomyelia. Radiology 118:609–111

144

CHAPTER 6

Musculoskeletal System: Girdles and Limbs

M. Bard, C. Massare, and S. Sintzoff

6.1 Applications

6.1.1 Present

For *tumours of bone and soft tissue,* CT enables differentiation between primary and metastatic lesions in anatomically complex regions such as the pelvis and the thigh. An intramedullary density difference of 20 HU between the limbs should lead us to check for a metastasis, but is not specific. Such a difference may result from infection, and clinical and pathological factors should be taken into account.

After diagnosis by conventional radiography, CT indicates the precise site of the lesion and its dimensions and volume. It shows the spatial extension of the lesion (endogenic or exogenic, superior or inferior) and determines whether it is limited or invasive. CT analyses the origin of the lesion and its relation to bony, vascular, nervous and muscular structures, and facilitates the performance of biopsy. The addition of contrast enhancement differentiates the vascular, necrotic and liquid components of a soft tissue tumour, and helps to define the extension of a primary bone lesion.

In the case of *infection,* CT effects the earliest diagnosis of acute osteomyelitis, by measuring the elevation of the attenuation coefficient of the marrow cavity (40–60 HU), and by detecting intramedullary gas. After a conventional diagnosis, persisting elevation of the attenuation coefficient is the sign of a subacute phase. Delineation of the involucrum and/or sequestrum and constriction of the medullary cavity by granulation tissue or dead bone are the signs of a chronic stage. During follow-up, CT allows differential diagnosis between healing—characterized by new bone formation on both sides of the cortex—and progression of the lesion. CT defines the extension of infection in the bone, the destruction of cortical bone and the extension in soft tissues with calcification. It may exclude a localized abscess and show the involvement of soft tissues, suggesting cellulitis and/or oedema.

In a general *anatomical, morphological examination,* a CT scan will define a congenital abnormality such as glenoid or acetabular dysplasia. A CT study plays a part in defining an acquired modification such as epiphysiolysis or aseptic necrosis of the tip.

As to *degenerative pathology,* CT is the method with which posterior coxarthrosis, transitory subluxation of the patella or trochlear chondropathy can be recognized earliest.

In *traumatic pathology,* thanks to its direct access without need of mobilization during the investigation, CT is helpful in the evaluation of comminuted fractures with luxation of shoulder or acetabulum. It can achieve primary diagnosis of a femoral head fracture, or after conventional radiography can define the precise configuration of the fracture and the localization of the fragments. CT defines the extension of an effusion or a haematoma in an articulation or in soft tissues, and is more effective than other methods in finding a sternoclavicular luxation or an osteochondral trochlear fracture.

Whatever the position of the lower limb might be, modified by dysplasia, arthrosis or infection, CT effects anatomical measurement of the anteversion angles of the acetabulum and femoral neck, as well as of the torsion of the inferior limbs. Finally, CT gives a better definition through the cast of the result of surgical reposition, of the acetabulum in congenital hip luxation in a child.

6.1.2 Future

CT is able to estimate the muscular atrophy and hypertrophy.

CT can measure the calcium content of the skeleton. Unlike other techniques, CT explores trabecular bone apart from cortical bone. Quantification of the trabecular bone may be effected by a specific apparatus used at a low energy rate, avoiding beam-hardening artefacts. The bone mineral content may be defined by Fourier image reconstruction and the dual source technique. There is a separate apparatus for measuring the calcium content of bone cortex and spongy bone in peripheral bone. Other methods are being elaborated.

The future applications of CT to the musculoskeletal system depend on the evolution of technology, but will include the study of the cruciate ligaments, the peripheral articulations and the small bones.

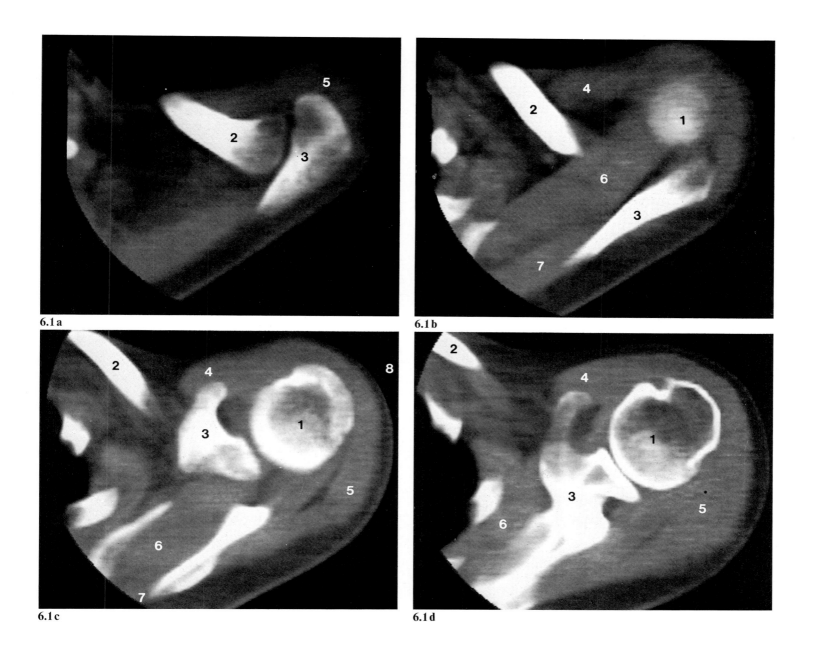

6.1 a

6.1 b

6.1 c

6.1 d

Fig. 6.1 a–d. Normal left shoulder. Differentiation of the muscular planes: **a** acromioclavicular level; **b** scapular spine level; **c** coracoïd level; **d** glenohumeral level.

1 Head of humerus
2 Clavicle
3 Scapula
4 Coracobrachialis muscle: short biceps

5 Deltoid muscle
6 Supraspinatus muscle
7 Angular rhomboïdeus muscle

147

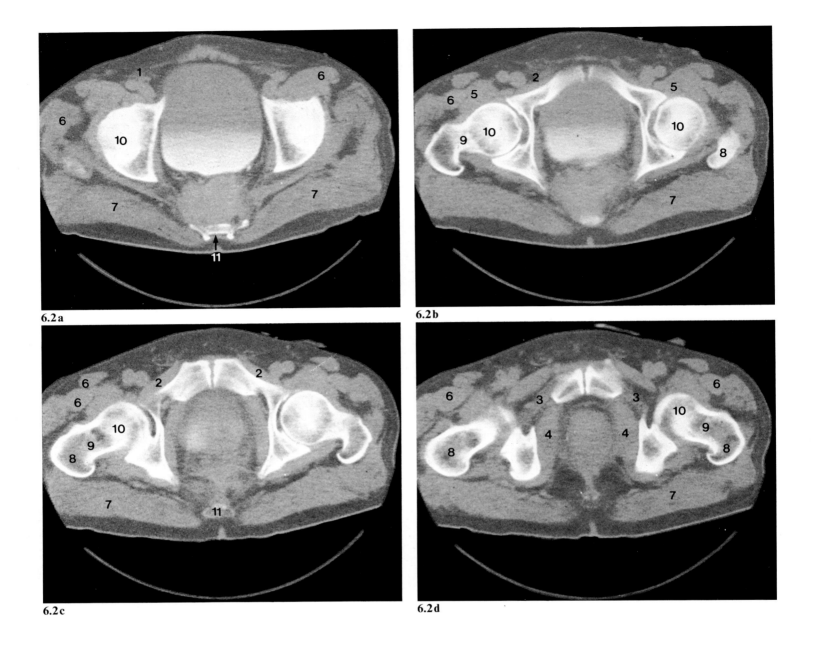

6.2a

6.2b

6.2c

6.2d

Fig. 6.2a–d. Normal coxofemoral articulation. Examination technique: The test should be effected in symmetrical dorsal decubitus; the feet are in neutral position. The sections should start at the level of the roof of the acetabulum and progress towards the lesser trochanter. The femoral head scan should follow the longest diameter of the head, allowing study of the relations with the acetabulum—the acetabular fossa and the anterior and posterior horns. Systematic study of the density of each femoral head reveals incipient necrosis, which is not visible on conventional radiography. Study of abduction and adduction reveals difficulty in movement of the femoral head and is used to check for head-acetabulum congruence before osteo-

tomy (reposition test). The sections are at the levels of **a** the roofs of the acetabula; **b** the femoral heads and the acetabular fossae; **c** the pubic symphysis and the junction between the femoral head and neck; **d** the neck and the greater trochanter.

1 Femoral vessels
2 Pectineal muscle
3 Obturator externus muscle
4 Obturator internus muscle
5 Psoas muscle
6 Triceps muscle
7 Gluteus muscle
8 Greater trochanter
9 Femoral neck
10 Femoral head
11 Coccyx

6.3 Musculoskeletal Tumours

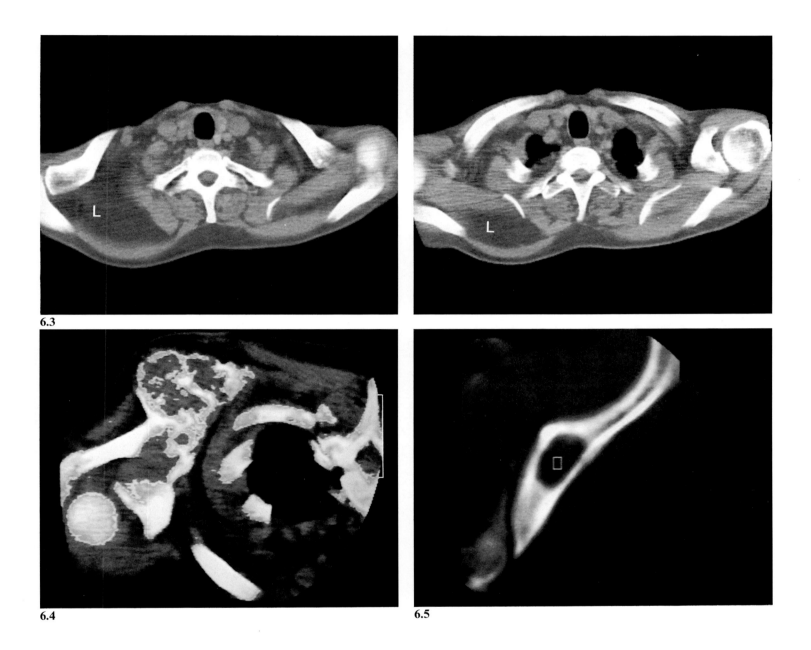

6.3

6.4

6.5

Fig. 6.3 Supraclavicular lipoma. There is a right, posterior, retro- and supraclavicular hypodense area (*L*) with a density of −120 HU, which is characteristic for fat. Muscle and bone structures are respected.
The usefulness of CT lies in revealing the nature of the lesion and in defining the locoregionl extension

Fig. 6.4. Scapular chondroma. The partly calcified tumoral process of the right scapula derives from the posterior bone cortex. Its border is regular and nearly complete. Note the lack of internal extension, e.g. towards the intercostal muscles and the ribs. Diagnosis was effected by biopsy. The advantage of CT is in demonstrating the potential for scapulectomy. There remains a cleavage plane, the thoracic muscles and bone structures being respected

Fig. 6.5. Eosinophilic granuloma of left ilium. This example of a benign pelvic tumour is seen here in a child. There is a centromedullary gap with a defined border, slightly narrowing the posterior bone cortex. Diagnosis was dubious on conventional radiological investigation

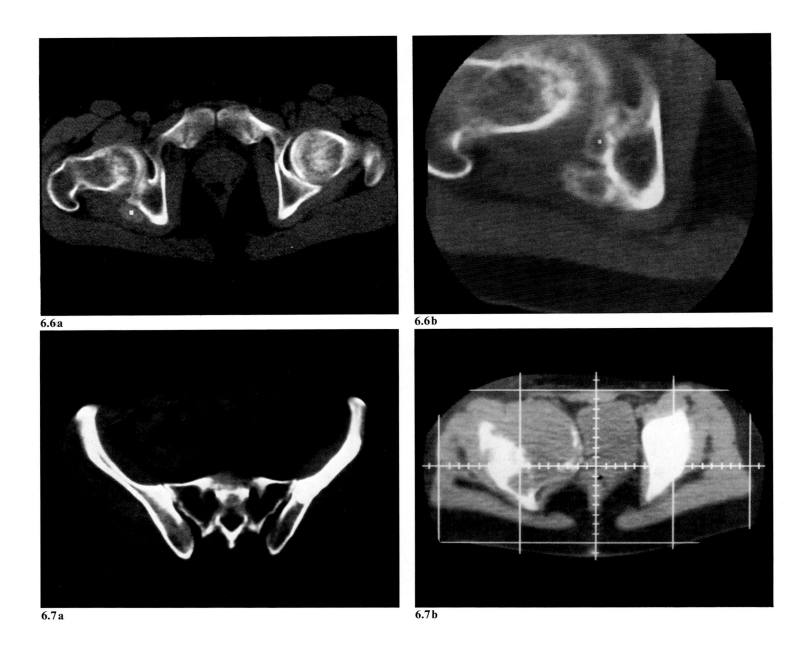

6.6a

6.6b

6.7a

6.7b

Fig. 6.7a, b. Chondroma of ilium. **a** Without extension.
Homogeneous density of the ilium; regular outlines; no locoregional extension; conventional radiography suspected the diagnosis, but cannot show whether there is extension into the soft tissues or not.
b With extension into soft tissue.
Spheroïd proliferation of the inferointernal outline of the right ilium with a calcified border, which is discontinuous but regular and presses back the bladder without infiltrations; diagnosis suspected on conventional radiological investigation.

The usefulness of CT is in defining the limits of the bone tumour, its volume, its eventual exopelvic and posterior extension, and especially its endopelvic, anterior extension with displacement or infiltration of the soft tissues

Fig. 6.6a, b. Calcifying myositis of the ischium. This example of a benign bone tumour in an adult displays contiguous tumefaction with a regular border. It is closely connected with the ischium without extension. Its density is compatible with an osteocartilaginous formation. **a** Total image; **b** detail of right hip 1 cm lower. Conventional investigations, including myelography and phlebography, were negative. Clinical sign: Incapacitating, recurring, right lumbosciatica. Surgical exploration of the lumbar disks L4–L5, L5–S was negative

150

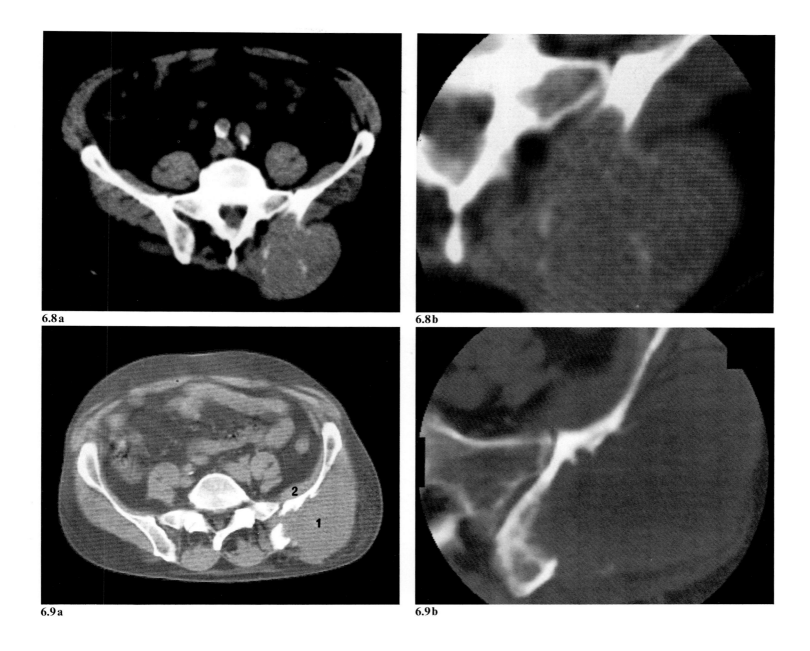

6.8a

6.8b

6.9a

6.9b

Fig. 6.8a, b. Osteosarcoma of ilium and ischium. **a** Total image. **b** Detail of left posterior iliac region. There is destruction of the posterior quarter of the ilium by an oviform tumefaction strewn with calcifications, which extends to the cutaneous plane without endopelvic involvement.

Conventional radiography was negative. Clinical sign: Painless tumefaction of the left gluteal area. CT defines the external extension and bone destruction, and shows precisely the limits of the endopelvic invasion

Fig. 6.9a, b. Chondrosarcoma of ilium and ischium. **a** Total image at L5 level. **b** Detail at S1 level. There is partial destruction of the left ilium and ischium with a soft proliferation (*1*) in the gluteal area and partial endopelvic extension (*2*).

The massive infiltration of the left gluteal muscles was known clinically. Conventional radiography is not very helpful. CT shows the exact topography of the gluteal tumefaction, the osteolysis and the endopelvic extension

151

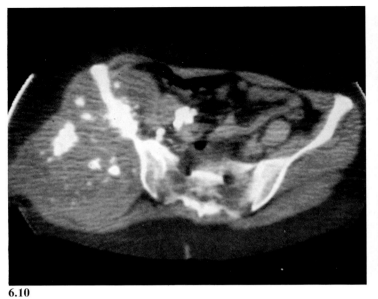

6.10

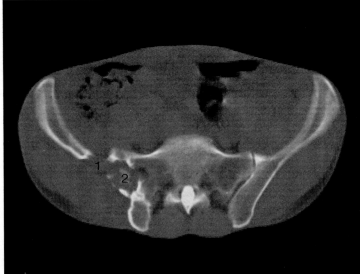

6.11a

6.11b

Fig. 6.10. Chondrosarcoma of ilium. Partial, irregular destruction of the right ilium is shown, with a calcified soft tissue proliferation and endo- and exopelvic extension into the overlying cutaneous area.
Diagnosis was by conventional radiography. CT exactly defines the extension not only into the gluteal muscles, but also into the pelvic cavity, helping the surgeon to reach the lesion more efficiently. It also facilitates differential diagnosis between osteochondroma and a chondrosarcoma.

The radiological characteristics of chondrosarcoma are:
Cartilaginous cuff of over 1 cm; denser centre; disorganized, heterogeneous ossification and calcification at some distance from the primary tumour

Fig. 6.11 a, b. Sacro-iliac chondrosarcoma. **a** Total image. **b** Detail of the right sacro-iliac region. There is destruction of the external part of the sacrum and the right ilium by a soft tumefaction (*1*) with a heterogeneous calcification invading the sacral foramen (*2*).

Conventional radiography, including myelography, was negative. Clinical sign: High truncal sciatica. In this case, thanks to its axial penetration, CT is the only method able to reveal the tumour of the sacrum

152

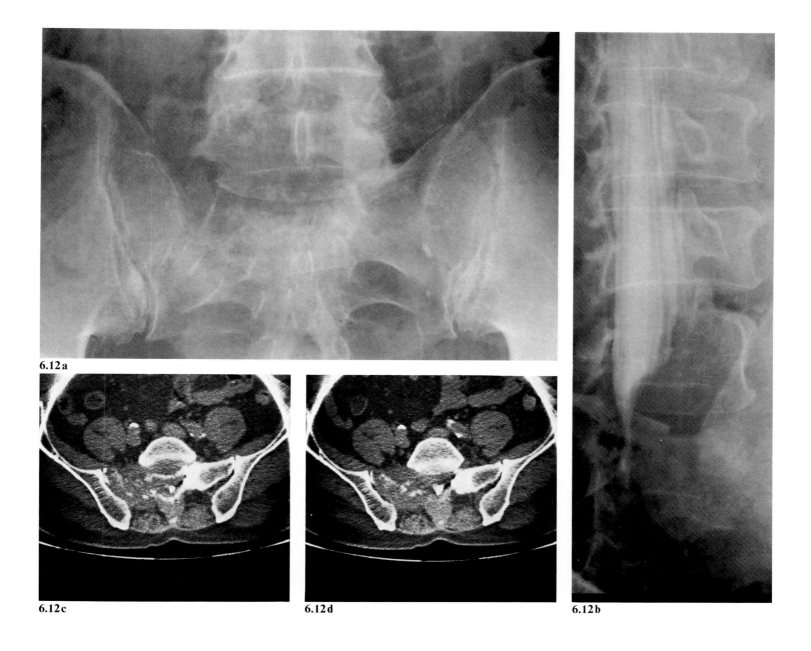

6.12a

6.12c   6.12d   6.12b

Fig. 6.12a–d. Lysis of sacrum. There is complete destruction of the right lateral with invasion of the posterior vertebral wall. Dense islets are present in the midst of the destructive process: this proliferation may accompany a chondrosarcoma.

Standard radiography suspected supero-extremal destruction of the right lateral mass of the sacrum. Myelography and tomographies showed extrinsic posterolateral, right compression at L5–S1, lysis of the posterior wall of S1 and the partially squeezed aspect of the anterior wall.

Clinical information: The patient had been treated for lung tuberculosis, and was sent to us with an atypical right lumbosciatica of the L4–L5 type with an S1 component. Biopsy in the sacral region indicated metastasis of a bronchial neoplasm. The pulmonary mass is known, considered as tuberculosis and treated as such. Multiple endoscopies were negative

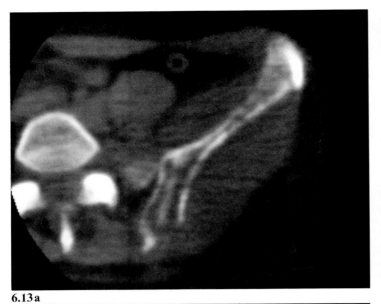

6.13 a

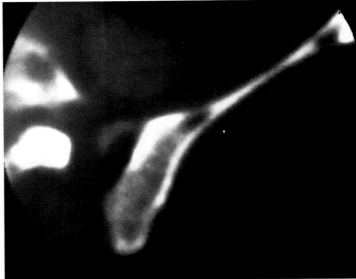

6.13 b

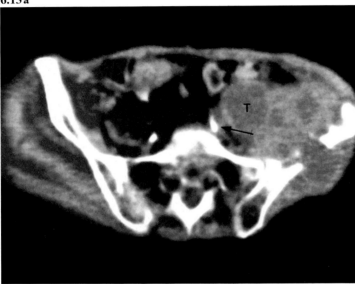

6.14

Fig. 6.13a, b. Iliac metastasis. **a** Permeative rarefaction of the external half of the left ilium, including trabecular and cortical bone: the morphology suggests a secondary lesion, confirmed by biopsy; diagnosis was neglected ovarian neoplasm. **b** Two areas of external and internal rarefaction; casual discovery during CT examination of the left hip; conventional radiography and scintigraphy normal; breast neoplasm 15 years previously.

CT facilitates early diagnosis of metastases in the pelvis

Fig. 6.14. Extensive iliac metastasis. A contrast-enhanced scan shows complete destruction of the medial third of the left ilium, with a soft proliferative extension of heterogeneous density (*T*) and exopelvic and (essentially) endopelvic backward displacement of the ureter (*arrow*). CT gives precise information on the extension of the tumoral area, not possible with conventional radiography

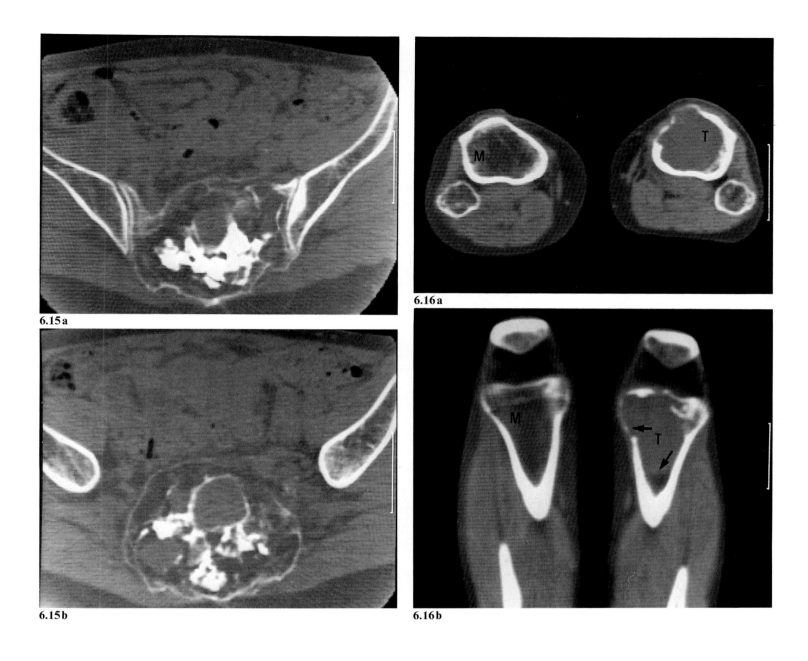

6.15a

6.15b

6.16a

6.16b

Fig. 6.15a, b. Giant cell tumour of sacrum. a A huge, heterogeneous tumour, involves the whole bone, with large zones of solid tissue and numerous calcifications. Note the absence of extension into the peritoneal soft tissues and the iliac bones. b A control scan 1 year later did not show any changes in this 60-year-old woman, 14 years after the first diagnosis and radiotherapy. The tumour is bordered by a narrow peripheral calcification without any rupture: this is only demonstrated by CT. This delicate shell is characteristic for either a giant cell tumour or an aneurysmal cyst

Fig. 6.16a, b. Giant cell bone tumour of left tibia. a Axial view. Note the cortical erosion, as seen on plain films, and also the involvement of the medullar cavity (M) by a soft tissue tumour (T): right, fat density; left, solid tumoral density. b Longitudinal view. This scan demonstrates not only the cortical erosion of the tibial plate and the internal cortex, but also the intramedullary extension of the soft tissue mass lower in the tibia

155

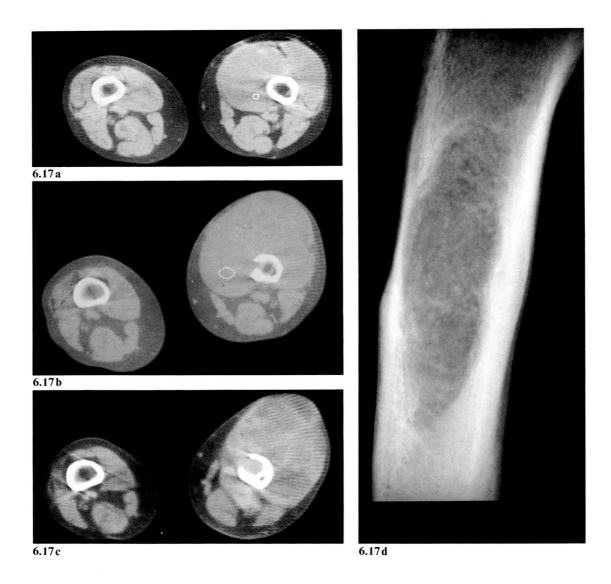

6.17a

6.17b

6.17c

6.17d

Fig. 6.17a–d. Evolution of rhabdomyosarcoma over 27 months. Diagnosis in this 65-year-old female patient was effected by means of a muscular biopsy in 1976. Amputation was refused. Radiotherapy was associated with several surgical debridements. **a** October 1979. Heterogeneous tumefaction involves the inferior third of the vastus medialis muscle group, as well as the anterior part of the rectus femoris muscle, without any involvement of the right femoral diaphysis. **b** December 1980. The tumour now involves the vastus lateralis muscle, abrading the femoral cortex. **c** January 1982. The bony extension has progressed into the medullary cavity, with para-endosteal osteogenesis. Contrast enhancement affords differentiation of the tumour in necrotic areas. The femoral artery is preserved, and there is no medullary extension upstream. **d** January 82. With conventional radiography, the penetration of the muscular tumour into the medullary cavity is less apparent

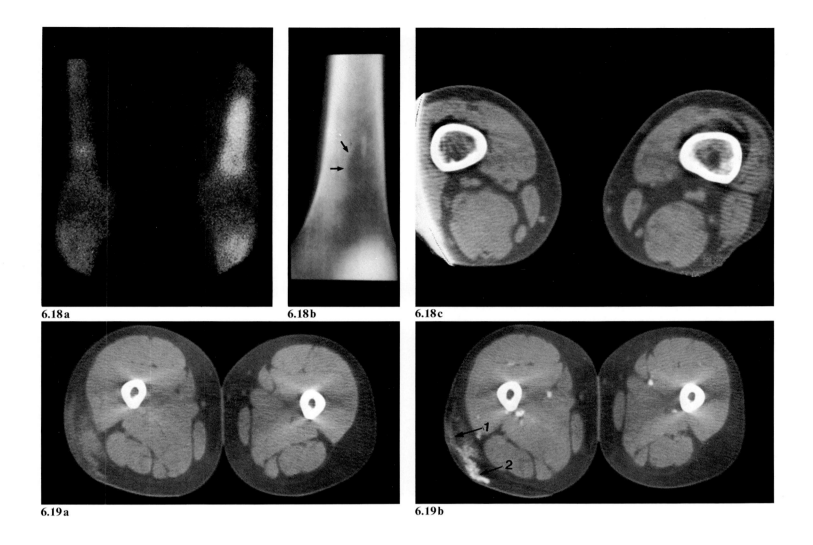

6.18a 6.18b 6.18c

6.19a 6.19b

Fig. 6.18a–c. Fat embolus in femur. **a** Isotopic scanning shows hyperfixation. **b** Conventional radiography, including tomography, demonstrates an egg-shaped, intraspongious area of bone rarefaction (*arrows*) in the inferior third of the femoral diaphysis, compatible with a fat infarction. **c** CT makes the diagnosis more precise: the rarefied density of the medullary bone is characteristic for fat.

Clinical information: There is a 3-month history of necrosis of the left femoral head. The patient is an alcoholic

Fig. 6.19a, b. Capillary angioma of thigh after embolization. **a** A plain scan reveals hyperdensity of the posterolateral fasciculation of the right thigh. **b** After rapid bolus injection of i.v. contrast material, an enhanced scan shows, in the soft tissues between the muscular planes and the subcutaneous plane, a capillary angioma (*1*) and a drainage vein (*2*).

The advantage of CT is that it is non-invasive. It demonstrates, in this case, that embolization was incomplete

157

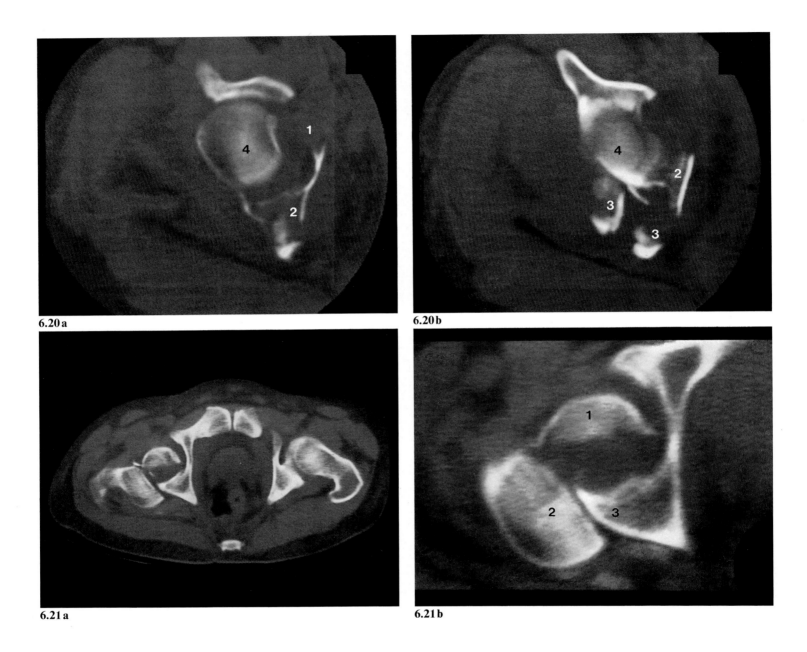

6.20a

6.20b

6.21a

6.21b

Fig. 6.20a, b. Parcelled fracture of acetabulum. **a** A scan of the femoral head (*4*), shows complete separation, through fracture, of the acetabular fossa with an endopelvic haematoma (*1*) and fracture of the posterior acetabular horn (*2*). **b** A scan of the superior part of the femoral head (*4*) reveals two posterior bone fragments (*3*).

Conventional radiography suspected a fracture of the acetabular fossa and the posterior horn. CT reveals and localizes the two posterior fragments and defines the fractures of the acetabular fossa and the posterior horn

Fig. 6.21a, b. Fracture of femoral head. **a** Total image. **b** Right hip detail, showing a fragment of the femoral head (*1*), a dislocated posterior fragment (*2*) and the posterior horn of the acetabulum. There is complete separation of the head by the posterior acetabulum horn, with posterior luxation of the posterior half of the head and the neck. Note the double posterior fragmentation inside a haematoma.

Conventional radiological investigations approached the diagnosis, but CT gives a precise image of the complete head separation and the luxation of its posterior half. Clinical information: The 22-year-old patient received dashboard injuries in a driving accident

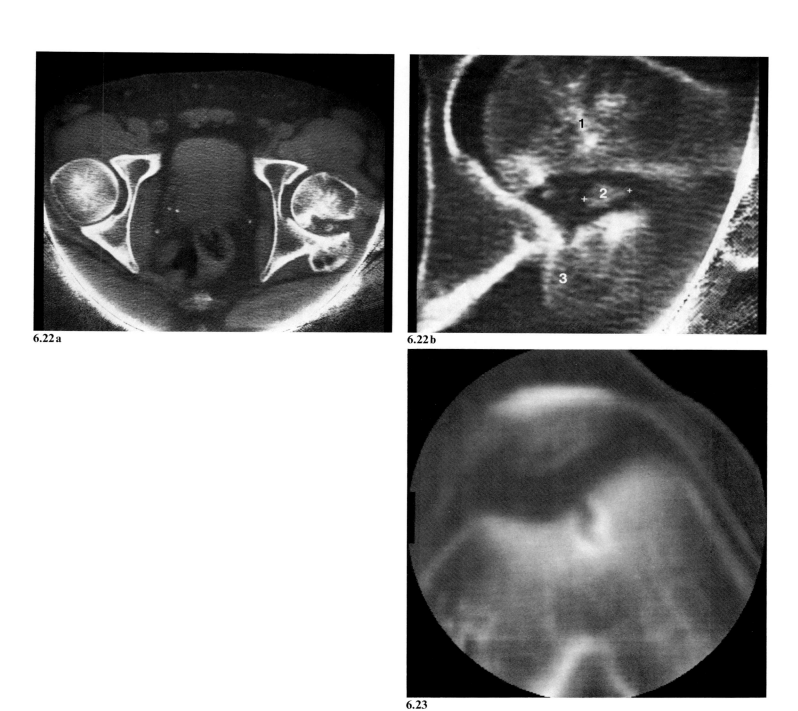

6.22a

6.22b

6.23

Fig. 6.22a, b. Old fracture of femoral head. **a** Scan of left and right hips. **b** Left hip detail, showing the femoral head (*1*), a 10-mm-long isolated fragment (*2*) and a posterior fragment of the head (*3*), which is incorporated into the posterior acetabular horn. The CT examination was made 1 year after the accident. The conventional radiographic examination, also 1 year after the accident, demonstrates a post-traumatic coxarthrosis (a consequence of an old acetabular fracture) and a luxation of the femoral head.

The major advantage of CT in acetabular trauma is the demonstration of femoral head fracture and articular fragmentation. Clinical information: The patient suffered dashboard injuries in a driving accident

Fig. 6.23. Osteochondral fracture of trochlear sulcus. CT demonstrated anteroposterior rupture when conventional radiography was negative. Clinical information: The patient received a direct shock against the dashboard in a traffic accident

159

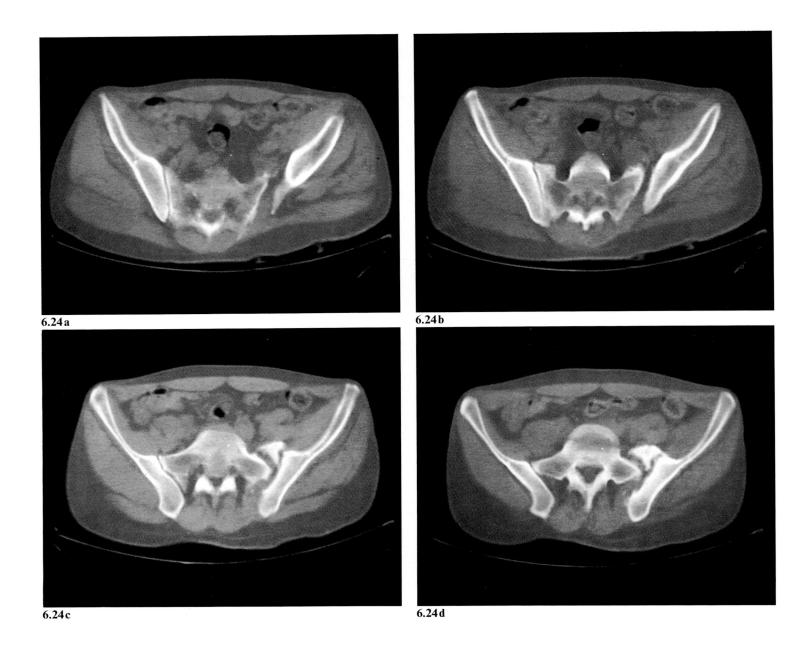

6.24a

6.24b

6.24c

6.24d

Fig. 6.24a–d. Sacro-iliac fracture-dislocation. **a, b** Plain scans demonstrating a left sacro-iliac luxation. **c** Plain scan revealing an oblique fracture of the left half of the sacrum. **d** Plain scan showing a small, endopelvic haematoma beneath a sacral fracture.

The sacral fracture was suspected on conventional radiography. The advantage of CT in emergency situations is to define, without any manipulation of the patient, the exact fracture type, the existence of a luxation and the change in the endopelvic soft tissues. Clinical information: The 30-year-old patient was involved in a traffic accident

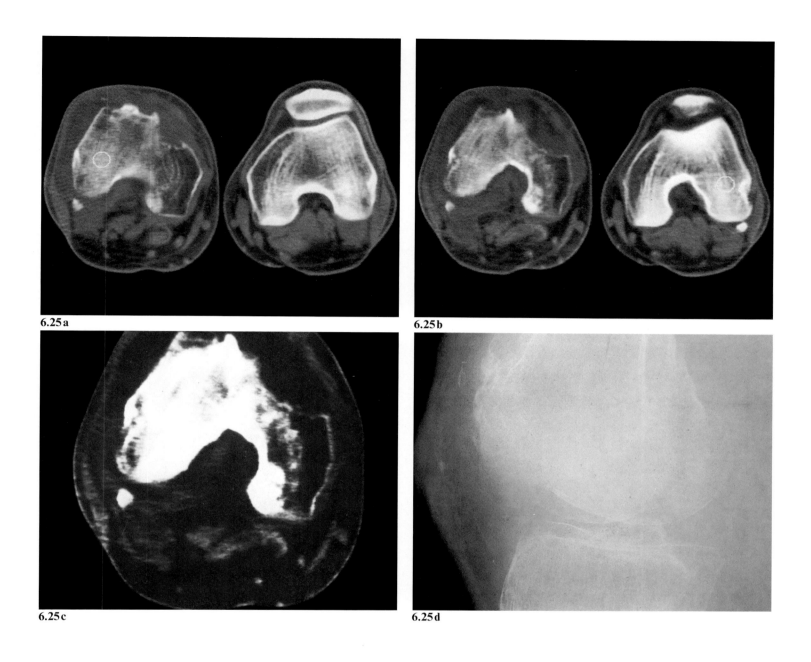

6.25a

6.25b

6.25c

6.25d

Fig. 6.25a–d. Compression fracture of trochlear sulcus. **a** Total image. **b** Total image 10 mm lower. **c** Magnification of right trochlear sulcus. **d** Conventional film of right knee in the lateral position.

Diagnosis was by conventional radiography. CT demonstrates loss of bone substance in the medial facet of the trochlear surface, with erosion and soft tissue swelling, and defines the compression depth of the medial surface. Clinical information: The examination was made 3 months after the accident; the patient had had patellectomy

161

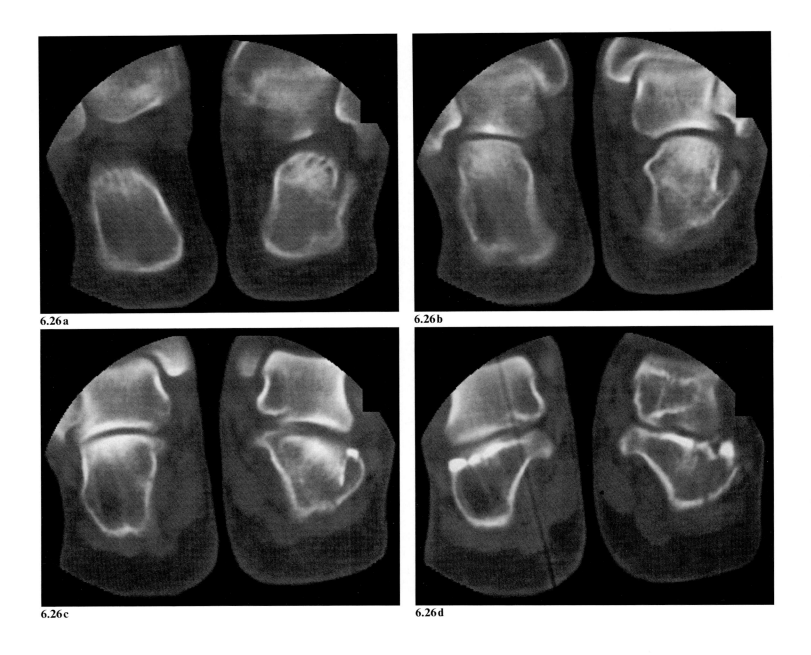

6.26 a

6.26 b

6.26 c

6.26 d

Fig. 6.26 a–d. Fracture of calcaneum: frontal study. **a** A section at the level of the posterior surface of the calcaneum shows a rupture of the superolateral cortex of the calcaneum. **b** A section at the level of the posterior third of the subtalar articulation reveals widening of the superolateral calcanean fracture. **c** A section at the level of the median third of the subtalar articulation demonstrates subsidence of the lateral half of the calcaneum with rupture of the inferolateral cortex. **d** A section at the level of the anterior third of the subtalar articulation shows a breach of the lateral third of the superior cortex of the calcaneum and an inferior rupture.

The specific advantage of CT in frontal study of the calcaneum is the precise analysis of the subtalar articulation and the vertical extension of the fracture

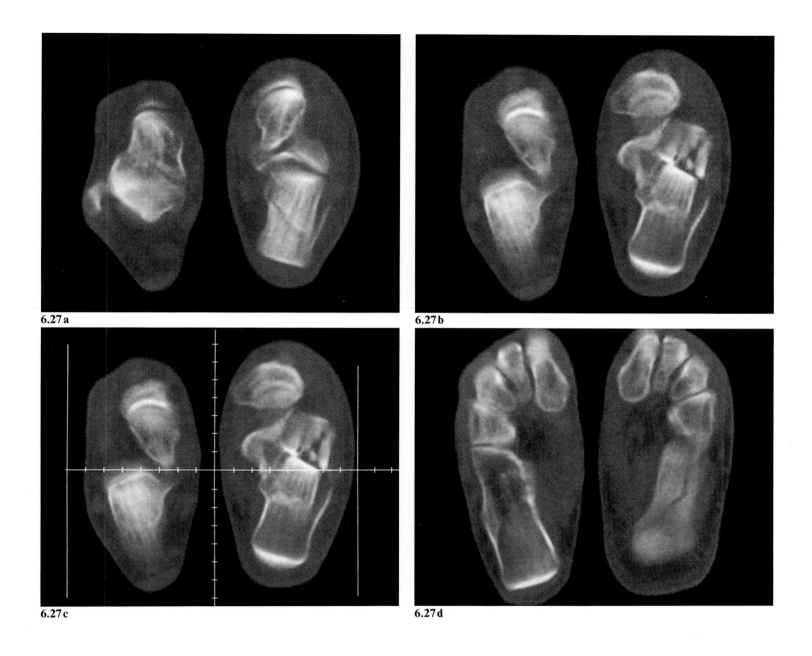

6.27 a

6.27 b

6.27 c

6.27 d

Fig. 6.27 a–d. Fracture of calcaneum: axial study. **a** A transverse section at the level of the subtalar articulation demonstrates an oblique fracture of the posterior surface of the calcaneum with a lateral, cortical rupture. **b** A section 10 mm under the subtalar articulation reveals a prethalamic, comminuted fracture of the calcaneum with a split at the back of the antero-internal surface. **c** A section at the same level with transverse and anteroposterior measurements. **d** A transverse section 20 mm under the subtalar articulation, at the level of the calcaneocuboid articulation. Note the longitudinal extension of the calcanean fracture.

CT defines the longitudinal and transverse extension of the fracture and its dimensional consequences. The major advantage of CT in fractures of the calcaneum is to allow axial and frontal exploration without any significant manipulation

163

6.5 Morphological Abnormalities

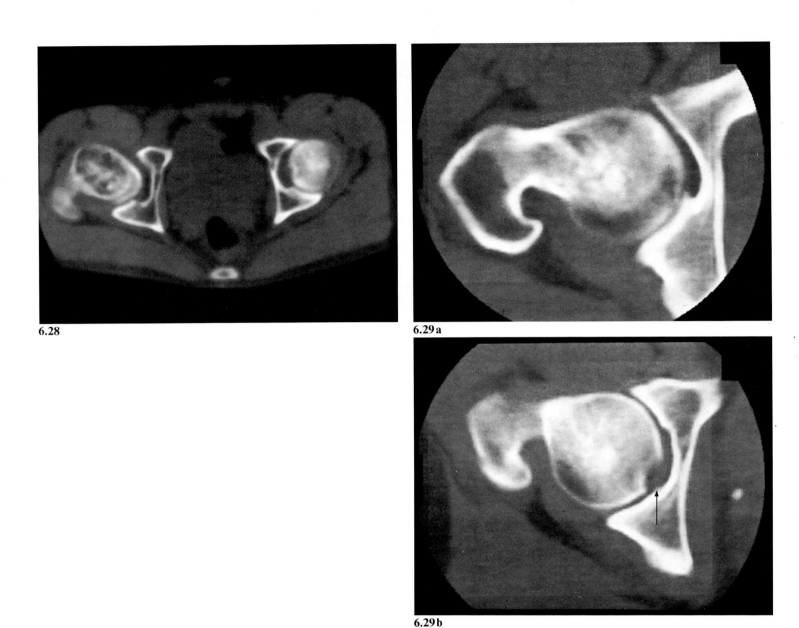

6.28

6.29 a

6.29 b

Fig. 6.28. Dysplastic hip. Egg-shaped deformity of the right femoral head is accompanied by bone rarefaction. The head-acetabulum incongruence causes lateral rotation.

The morphological diagnosis was effected by conventional radiography. The contribution of CT is the axial demonstration of a femoral head dysplasia; it reveals, moreover, a hypoplasia of the anterior acetabular horn, which increases the articular incongruity

Fig. 6.29a, b. Acquired coxopathy due to epiphysiolysis. **a** Neutral position. The scan shows deformity of the head with retroversion, and anteposition of the neck. **b** Dynamic test in medial rotation. The head hooks onto an osteophyte (*arrow*).

The morphological diagnosis was established by conventional radiography. The specific advantage of CT is that it defines the malposition of head and neck; it also reveals an osteophyte in the acetabular fossa

6.6 Articular Lesions

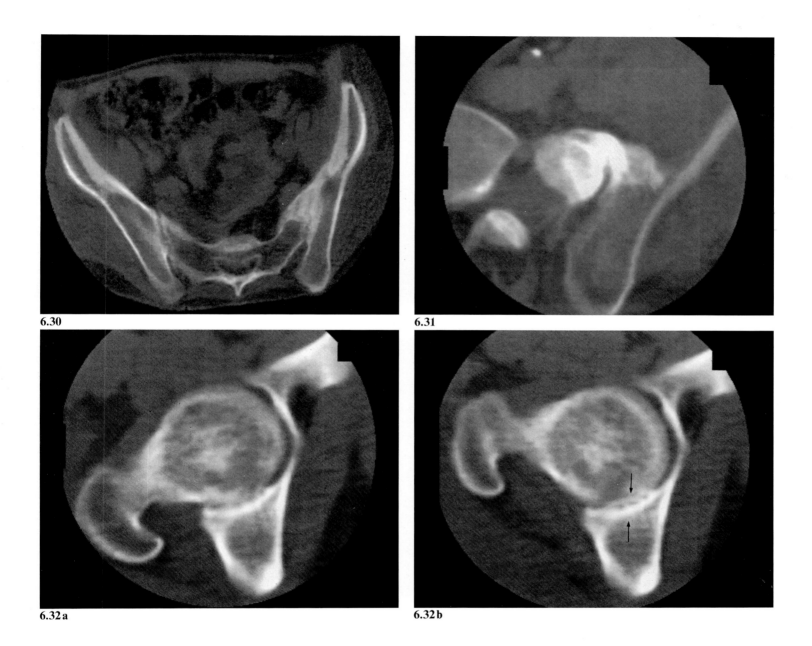

6.30

6.31

6.32 a

6.32 b

Fig. 6.30. Condensing arthrosis with Paget's disease of the bone. Corticospongious dedifferentiation of the anteromedial outline of the ilium is especially evident on the left. Note also condensation of the margins of the narrowed sacro-iliac articulations with synostosis on the left. Diagnosis was by conventional radiography. C.T. gives a precise evaluation of the extension of the lesion

Fig. 6.31. Sacro-iliac arthrosis based on a transitional anomaly. There is narrowing of the anterior third of the left sacro-iliac articulation, with condensation of the margins and geodes but without erosion. Diagnosis was effected by conventional radiography. The specific advantage of CT is the precise axial localization of the degenerative modification

Fig. 6.32a, b. Posterior coxarthrosis. **a** Lateral rotation; **b** medial rotation. The scans show posterior narrowing of the cartilage with a sinuous acetabular condensation (*arrows*). Dynamic study allows visualization of the posterior hooking of the head with the acetabular fossa. Conventional investigations, including coxometry, false profile and arthrography, were negative.

Clinical information: This 32-year-old patient had unexplained painful coxopathy

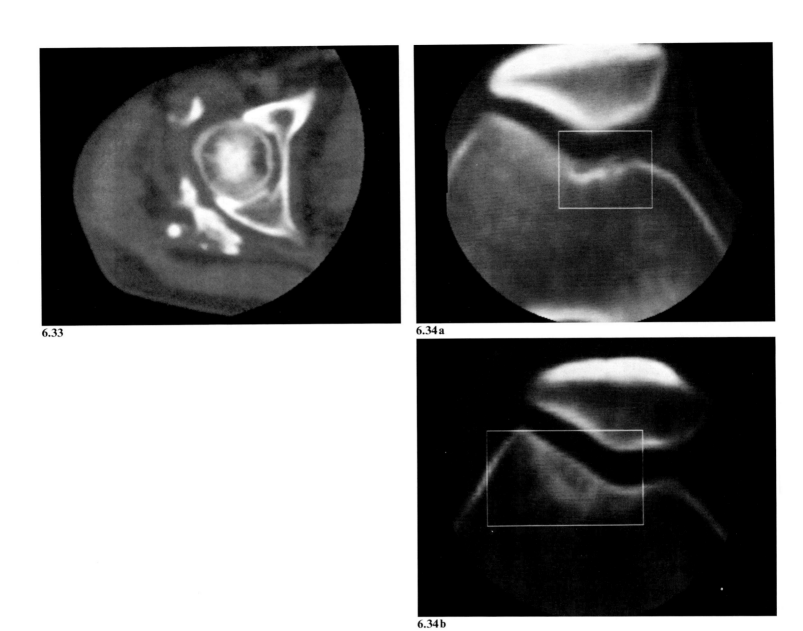

6.33

6.34a

6.34b

Fig. 6.34a, b. Chondromalacia of trochlear surface of femur. a Medial facet. There is sclerotic subchondral depression with residual penetration. b Lateral facet. The subchondral osteolysis has a sclerotic border in the deeper part. Conventional radiography, including tomography and arthrography, was negative. Clinical information: These two young patients had chronic knee pain

Fig. 6.33. Periarthritis of hip. CT detail of the right hip demonstrates pericapsular, anterior and posterior calcifications. These lesions were suspected on conventional radiography but only CT permits precise localization of the calcifications in regard to the articulation

6.7 Aseptic Necrosis

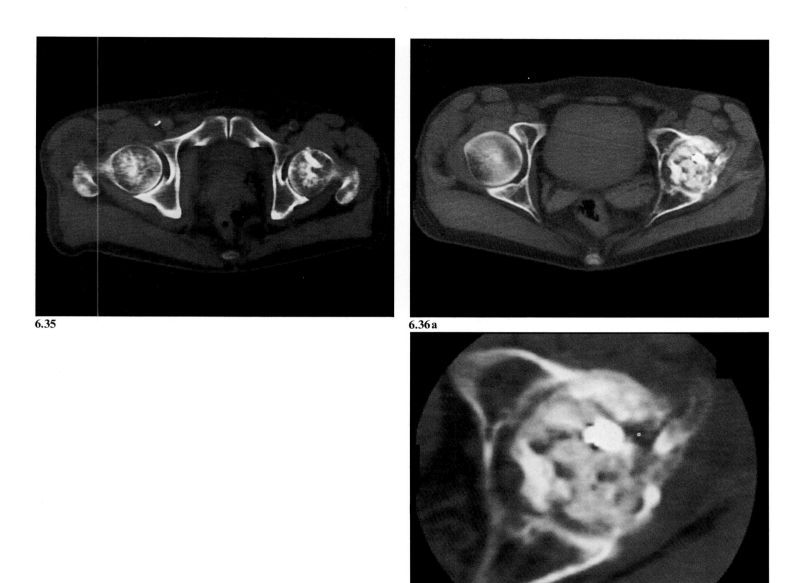

6.35

6.36a

6.36b

Fig. 6.35. Early necrosis of left femoral head. A plain scan of the hips shows narrowing of the bone cortex, reduction of the trabecular distribution and anterior densification in the midst of a rarefaction area. These modifications were not apparent on conventional radiography. The advantage of C.T. is in diagnosing incipient necrosis earlier than conventional methods. Comparison of the densities of the two femoral heads gives a control of the contralateral hip. Moreover, in cases of lacking articular congruity, CT enables dynamic recentering tests

Fig. 6.36a, b. Aseptic necrosis. **a** Total image; **b** detail of left hip. The whole structure of the femoral head is modified. The spongious bone is transformed into multiple small islands of necrotic bone with a high, variable density, separated by rarefied areas, and the cortex is broken up, e.g. on the posterior and anterolateral surfaces.
The diagnosis was evident on conventional radiography, but CT gives a better representation of the extension of necrosis, as well as allowing a control of the contralateral hip. Demonstration of the exact topography is helpful in the pre-operative work-up

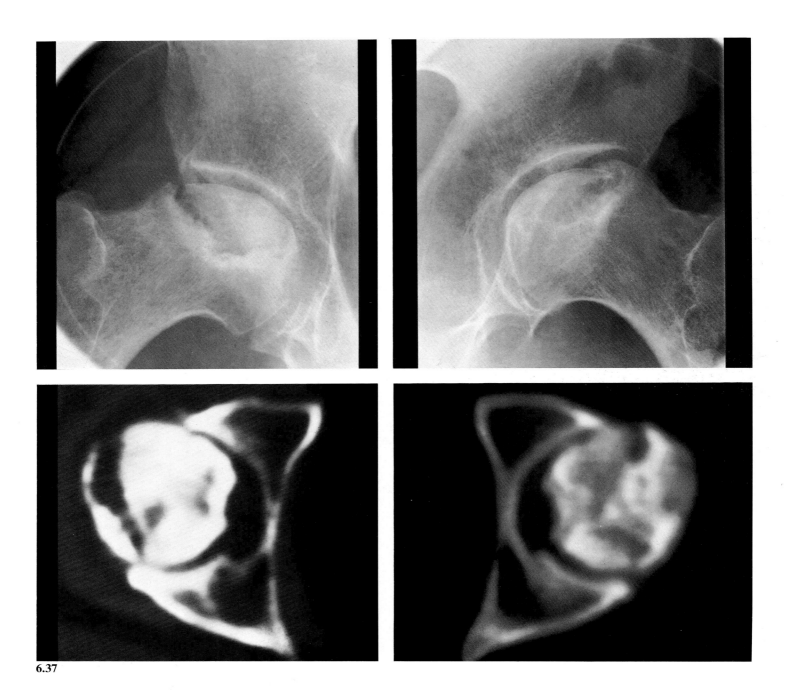

Fig. 6.37. Bilateral aseptic necrosis. *Above:* conventional radiography. *Below:* CT at upper femoral head level. On CT the cortical separation of the external third is seen to involve the whole right femoral head. The anteroposterior, median cortical disinsertion of the left femoral head cannot be estimated by conventional methods.

Clinical information: The necrosis was detected a year before in a 37-year-old patient without any traumatic or professional antecedents

and without any history of relevant disease, corticotherapy or alcoholism.

Based on the conventional radiographic examination, the surgeon had proposed bilateral derotation of the femoral heads. The demonstration by CT of the precise extension of the sequestration led to postponement of the operation

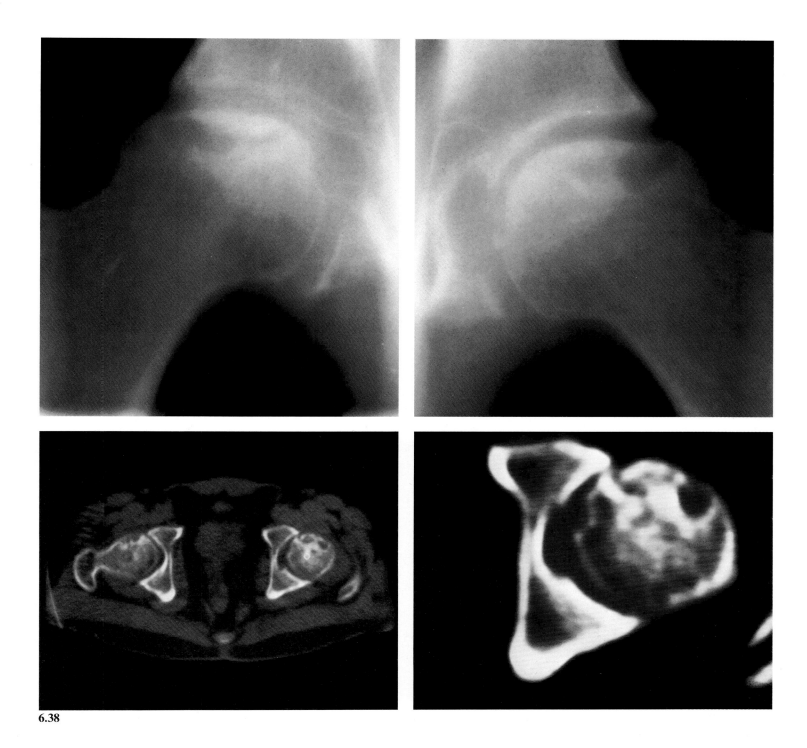

6.38

Fig. 6.38. Bilateral aseptic necrosis. *Above:* conventional radiography showing a bilateral supero-external depression. *Below:* total image (*right*) and left hip detail (*left*).
The cortical disinsertion and necrotic densification are only found in the anterior part of each femoral head.

The specific advantage of CT is once more to define the limits of the lesion, which in this case is only anterior, without any extension, in contrast to the case illustrated in Fig. 6.37. Clinical information: The patient was 45 years old. The diagnosis was made 10 months previously after 8 months corticotherapy

169

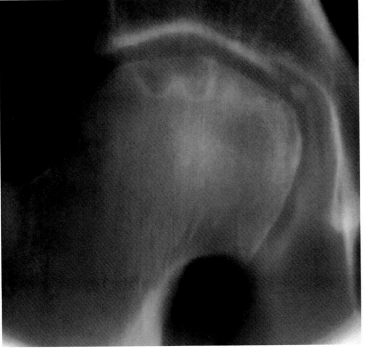

6.39 a

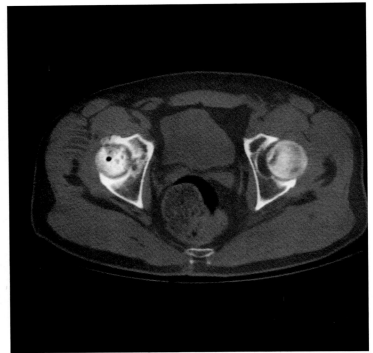

6.39 b

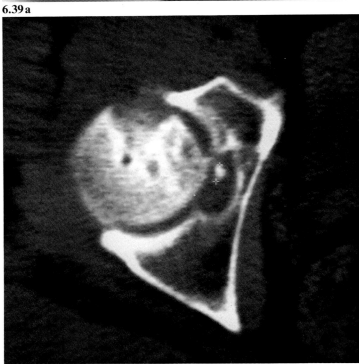

6.39 c

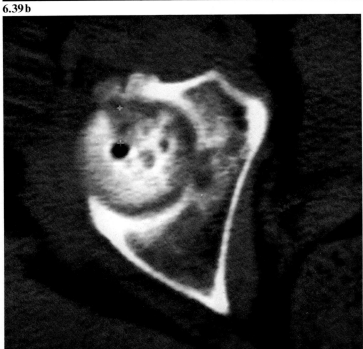

6.39 d

Fig. 6.39 a–d. Aseptic necrosis. **a** Conventional tomography of the right hip shows general collapse of the superior outline of the femoral head, with an isolated bone fragment at the back of the acetabulum, proving a mature aseptic necrosis. Note the beginning of the cartilage-narrowing process at the union of the roof and fossa of the acetabulum. **b** CT of both hips. CT confirms the existence of the isolated fragment of the anterior part of the acetabular fossa. **c** Section in the middle third of the right femoral head. **d** Section in the upper third of the right femoral head. CT also reveals another isolated fragment beginning at the line of union of the anterior and medial parts of the femoral head. It also objectifies, an irregular thickening of the anterior acetabular horn, which may have a traumatic origin.

It shows the extension of the destruction of the femoral head, which is triangular in its anterior part and notched in the central part, and elicits a paracentral air bubble in the head.

The advantage of CT is that it details the extension of the necrotic process, not only in the anterior part of the head, but also in the central area. It shows early cortical fragmentation, not revealed by conventional radiography. It visualizes, moreover, a probable post-traumatic state of the anterior part of the acetabulum, which may be an etiological factor of the bone disease.

Clinical information: This was casual discovery in a patient aged 51 who consulted because of chronic pain in the right knee. Arthrography revealed chondromalacia of the internal patellar surface with fissuration

170

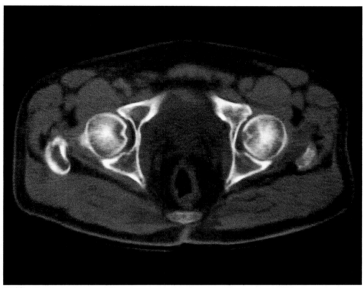

6.40a

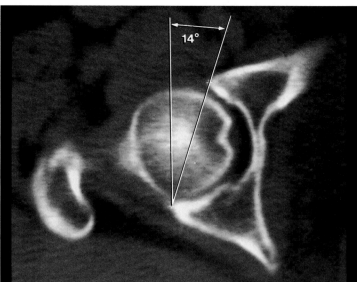

6.40b

6.40c

Fig. 6.40a–c. Anteversion angle of the acetabulum. **a** Total image; **b** detail of right hip; **c** detail of left hip.

The examination is performed with the patient in symmetrical dorsal decubitus with the feet in the neutral position. The symmetry of the femoral heads is controlled by a global scan: the tangent to the posterior outline of the femoral heads, which represent the pelvic axis, should be perpendicular to the anteroposterior axis. The measurements are made on the section where the head displays its greatest diameter and where both acetabular horns are seen. The angle of horizontal acetabular anteversion is the angle between the line perpendicular to the pelvis axis (VP) and the line tangential to the anterior and posterior acetabular horns (AP). The normal range is 15°–20°.

The major indications are: Congenital luxation due to acetabular dysplasia: the angle is increased in anterior insufficiency and is reduced in posterior insufficiency; Protrusive coxarthrosis due to malformation of the acetabulum in retroversion with neck retroversion and coxa vara; Post-traumatic, and postsurgical follow-up

171

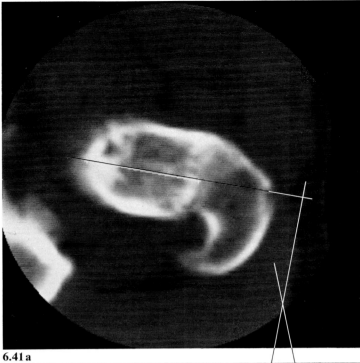

6.41 a

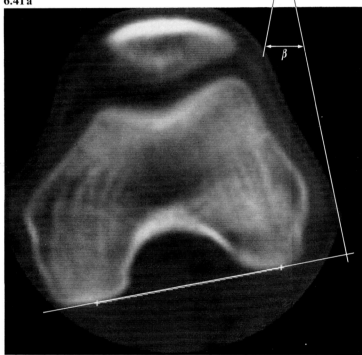

6.41 b

Fig. 6.41 a, b. Anteversion angle of the femoral neck. The anteversion angle is the angle between the perpendicular to two planes: **a** The neck axis. The exact section of the neck plane is shown by parallelism between the anterior and the posterior margins (not between the centre of the femoral head and the centre of the neck, because in normal anatomical conditions the head can be displaced relative to the neck axis). **b** The tangent to the bicondylar plane, taken from the section where the maximum expansion of the condyles is seen.

The normal values are 25° in children and 5°–15° in adults. The patient lies in symmetric dorsal decubitus with the feet in the neutral position.

CT is more precise than conventional radiography (error from 5% to 30%) in calculating the angle, but the conventional approach is more practical. CT should be performed if the angle is greater than 30° if there is a surgical indication.

Orthopaedic Interest in the Anteversion Angle. The determination of the anteversion angle is useful in congenital luxation and the pathogeny of rotation abnormalities of the inferior limbs. A persisting anteversion angle during childhood results first in an inward rotation of the femurs, with the feet turned inwards, and later in a correction with the feet turned outwards. The outcome is a double torsion: an inward rotation of the femur and an outward rotation of the tibia.

A modification of the anteversion angle interferes in the pathogeny of arthrosis. It is well known that in the frontal plane coxa vara or coxa valga may induce arthrosis. In the transverse plane, a coxa valga is often associated with an anteversion, a coxa vara with a retroversion. A possible origin of essential coxarthrosis is coxa retrorsa.

Knowledge of the anteversion angle is necessary before a Pauwels osteotomy and detorsion. Study of the anteversion angle is indicated in post-traumatic evaluation. A pertrochanteric fracture usually involves a retroversion by outward rotation of the femur, under the action of the gluteus medius muscle. As a result of the knee position during the operation, nailing of the femur with a closed focus leads to either anteversion, if the patella is at the zenith, or retroversion, if the leg is in a position of outward rotation

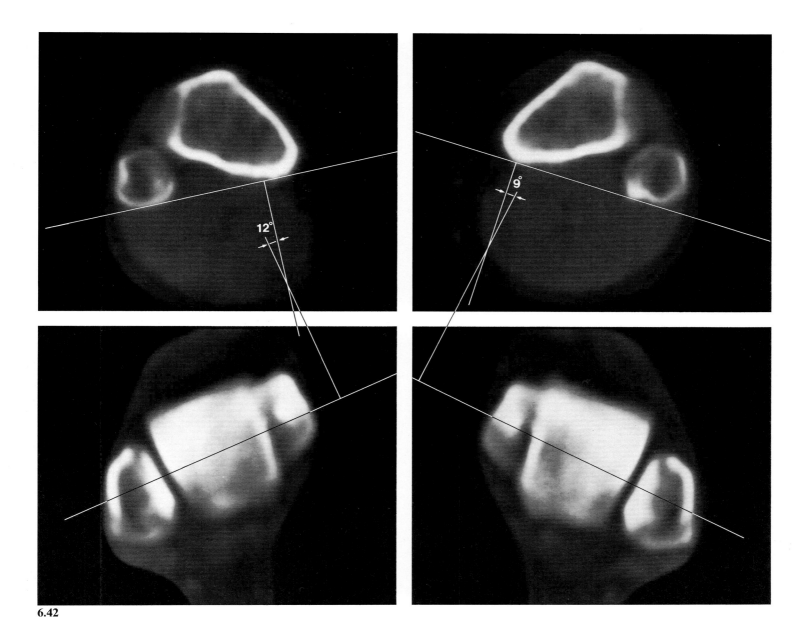

6.42

Fig. 6.42. Lateral tibial torsion. The angle of tibial torsion is the angle formed by the intersection of the lines perpendicular to: (a) the tangent to the posterior margins of the tibia and fibula on a scan of the superior fibulotibial articulation and (b) the transverse axis of the tibiotarsal articulation on a section at the level of the upper surface of the talus. The patient lies in decubitus with symmetrical extension of the lower limbs. The position of the feet is neutral.

Pathology: 1. Lateral torsion of the tibia may be determined by abnormal anteversion of the neck, primary lateral torsion of the diaphysis and chronic lateral subluxation of the patella. 2. Medial tibial torsion exists when the angle is below 15°

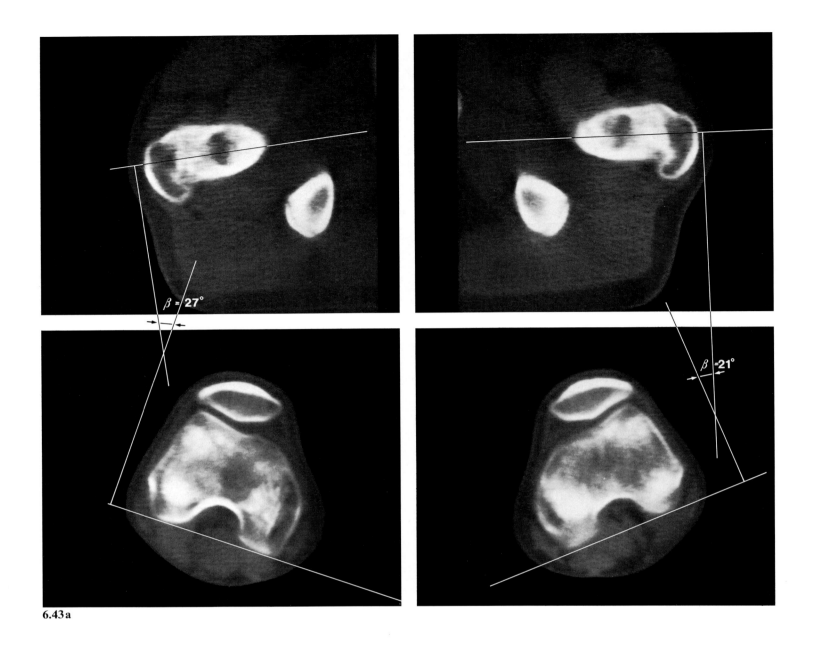

6.43a

Fig. 6.43a, b. Global study of torsion of inferior limbs in a case of right lateral tibia torsion. The torsion is evaluated by measuring the anteversion angle of each femoral neck and the angle of tibial torsion. The specific advantage of CT is that it gives a precise, anatomical calculation of the torsion of the inferior limbs, whatever their position, when modified by dysplasia or arthrosis. **a** Anteversion angle of the femoral neck. **b** Torsion angle of the tibia

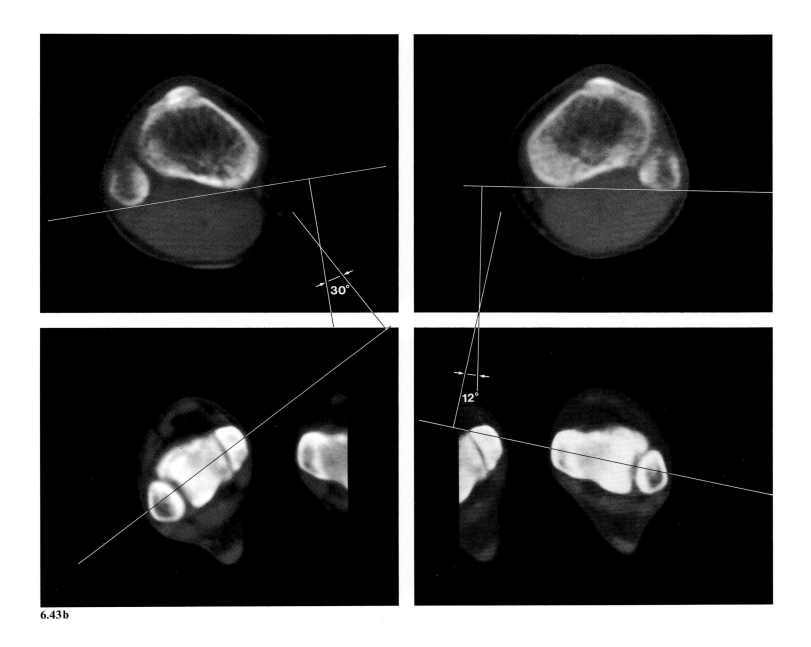

6.43b

175

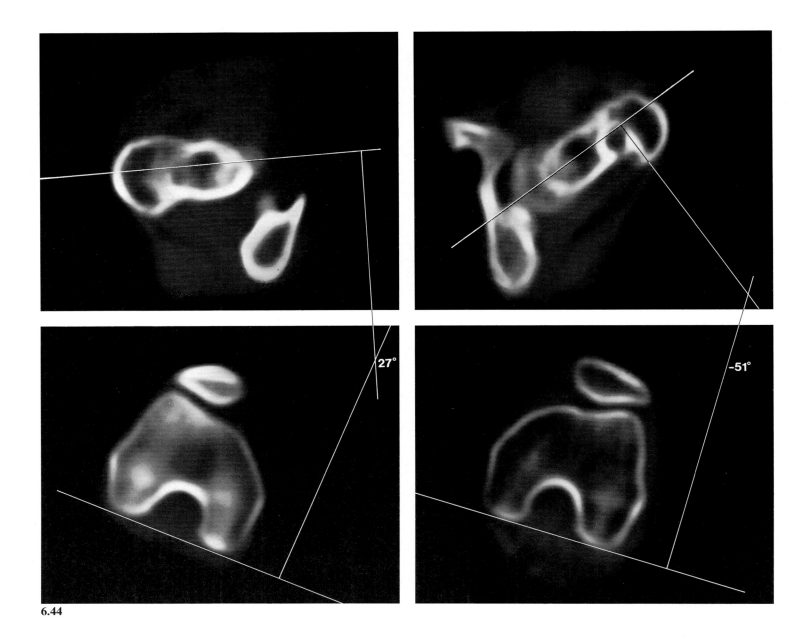

27°

−51°

6.44

Fig. 6.44. Iatrogenic torsion anormaly. A mediodiaphyseal femur fracture at the age of 18 years was treated by centromedullary nailing maintained for 20 months. After consolidation there was a 25-mm shortening and on outward torsion of the distal fragment, measured clinically at 45°.

CT reveals retroversion of the left femoral neck of −21°, compared with 27° on the right, provoking outward rotation of the distal femur and the tibia. The scan illustrates the necessity of a rigorous orthopaedic technique; ideally, torsion should be measured before and after centromedullary nailing

176

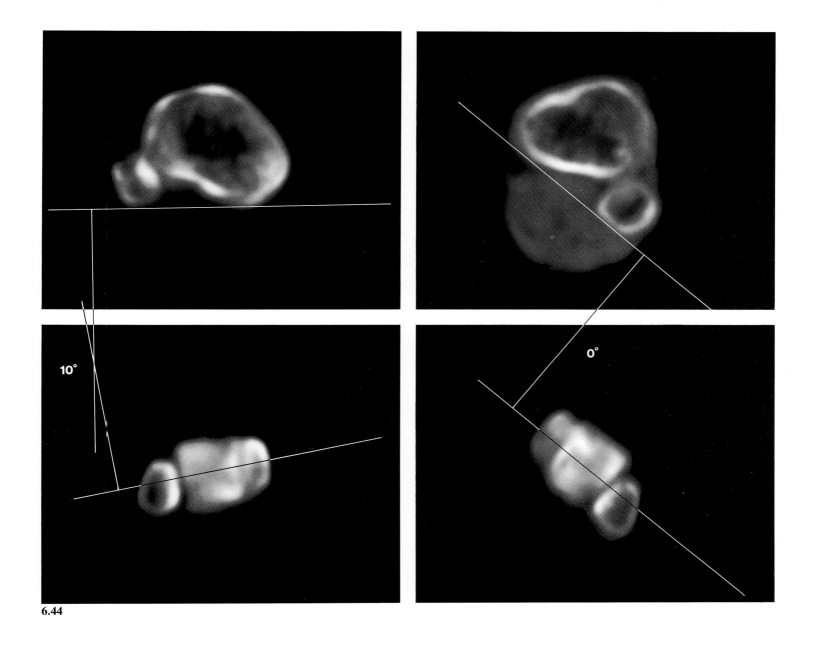

6.44

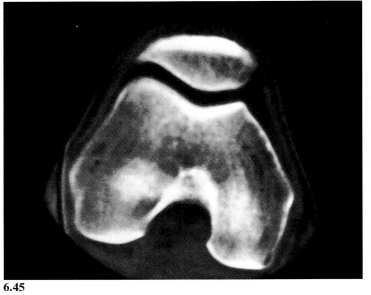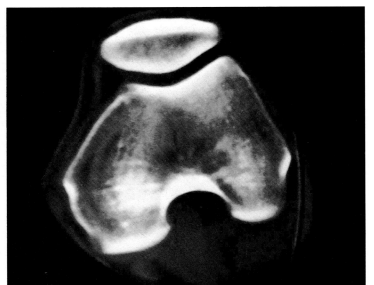

6.45

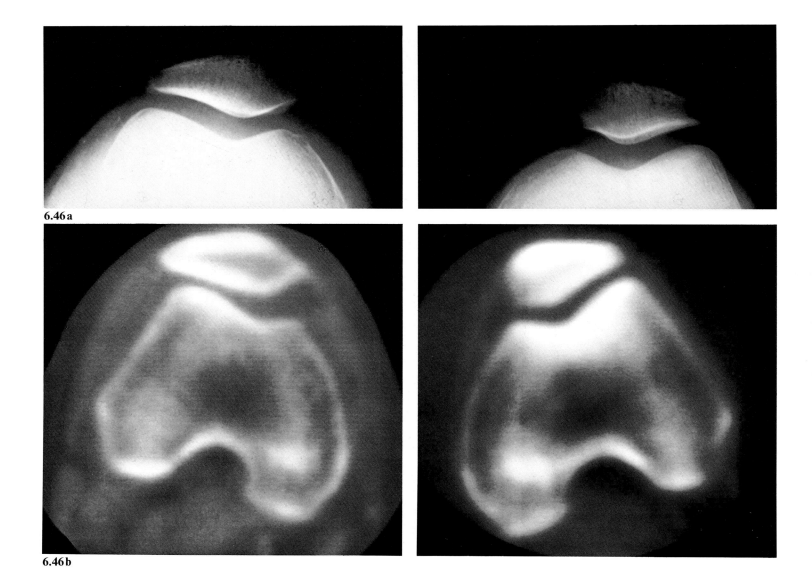

6.46 a

6.46 b

178

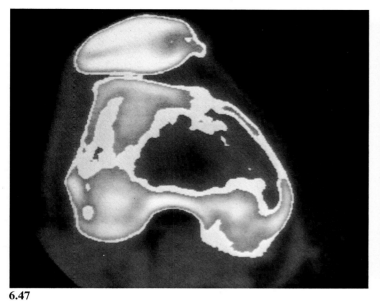

6.47

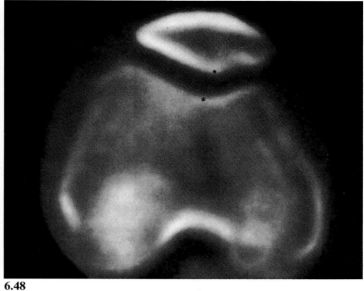

6.48

Fig. 6.47. Iatrogenic disorder of patella after section of lateral retinaculum. This hypocorrection is associated with a lateral articular narrowing and hyperpressure

Fig. 6.48. Iatrogenic disorder of patella after section of lateral retinaculum. This hypercorrection is associated with medial subluxation with erosion of the medial facet of the patella and chondropathy. The patella was normal before surgery

◁ **Fig. 6.45.** Normal entrance of the patella. In normal morphology of the patella and trochlea threre is congruity between them and a regular joint line. The patient is in decubitus position with knees fixed in 15° flexion and feet immobilized in the neutral position. A first scan is effected without any quadriceps contraction, a second (after measuring the distance TS-AT) with contraction of the quadriceps. The first 20° of flexion correspond to the functional entrance of the patella into the trochlear sulcus.

The specific contribution of CT is to reveal any temporary pathological subluxation at the moment of entrance, which cannot be found by conventional radiography

Fig. 6.46a, b. Temporary patellofemoral subluxation. **a** Conventional radiography with the knees in 30° flexion demonstrates normal patello-femoral joints. **b** CT with the knees in 15° flexion diagnoses subluxation of the right patella with narrowing of the external articular space.

This is an example of the specific usefulness of CT for the diagnosis of a transitory, pathological subluxation in the entrance sector, which cannot be approached by conventional radiography

179

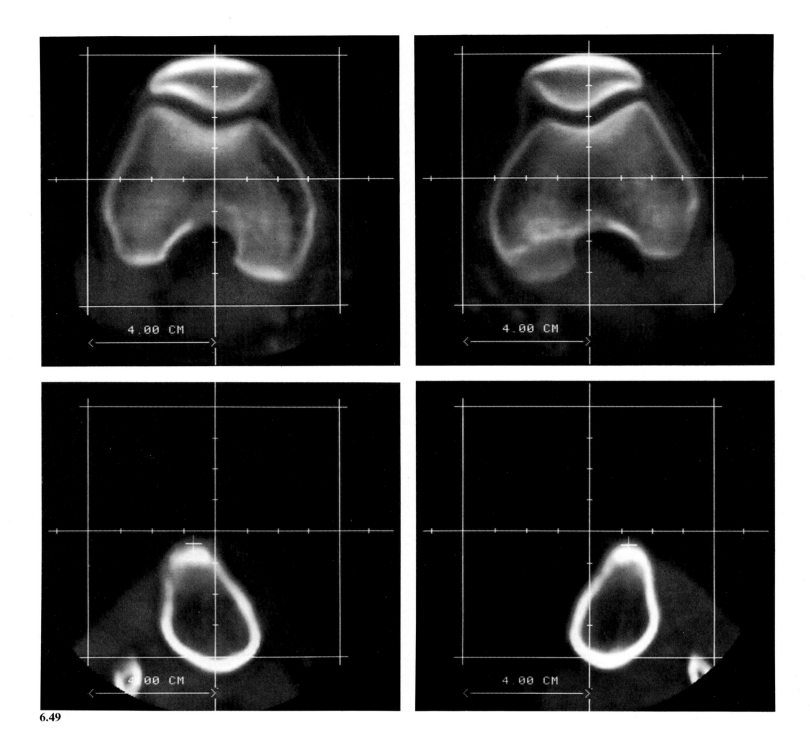

Fig. 6.49. Measurement of the distance between the trochlear sulcus and the tibial tubercle. This distance is calculated directly using two perpendiculars, one toward the trochlear sulcus, the other toward the tibial tubercle. The normal range is from 8 to 15 mm in the lateral position.

Measurement is made during the study of the patellofemoral articulation with 15° flexion, before the contraction of the quadricipital muscles. The upper section is realized in the plane of the trochlear sulcus, the lower one in the plane of the tibial Tubercle. The advantage of CT is its precision, permitting evaluation before and after surgical transplantation of the tubercle

180

References

1. Archer CR, Yeager V (1978) Internal structures of the knee visualized by computed tomography. J Comput Assist Tomogr 2:181–133
2. Bard M, Massare C, Busson J (1978) Indications du scannographe ou tomodensitometre corps entier en pathologie osteo-articulaire. Actual Rhuma 15:248–252
3. Bernardino ME, Jing BS, Thomas JL, Lindell MMS, Zornoza J (1981) The extremity soft-tissue lesion: A comparative study of ultrasound, computed tomography, and xereradiography. Radiology 139:53–59
4. Borlaza GS, Seigel R, Kuhns LR, Good AE, Rapp R, Martel W (1981) Computed tomography in the evaluation of sacroiliac arthritis Radiology 139:437–440
5. Carrera GF, Foley WD, Kozin F, Ryan E, Lawson TL (1981) CT of sacroiliitis. AJR 136:41–46
6. Delgado-Martins H (1979) A study of the position of the patella using computerised tomography. J Bone Joint Surg [Br] 61(4):443–444
7. Despontin J, Thomas P (1978) Reflexions sur l'etude de l'articulation femoro-rotulienne par la methode des tomographies axiales transverses computerisees. Acta Orthop Belg 44:857–870
8. Destouet JM, Gilula LA, Murphy WA, Sagel SS (1981) Computed tomography of the sternoclavicular joint and sternum. Radiology 138:123–128
9. Dihlmann W, Guertler KF, Heller M (1979) Sakroiliakale Computertomographie. Rofo 130:659–665
10. Dunnick NR, Brooks RA, Welch MS (1981) Abstracts of articles on computed tomography from non-radiological journals. J Comput Assist Tomogr 5:451–455
11. Egund N, Ekelund L, Sako M, Persson B (1981) CT of soft-tissue tumors. AJR 137:725–729
12. Fagan CS, Schreiber MH, Amparo EG, Wysong CB (1979) Traumatic diaphragmatic hernia into the pericardium: Verification of diagnosis by computed tomography. J Comput Assist Tomogr 3:405–408
13. Ginaldi G, de Santos LA (1980) Computed tomography in the evaluation of small round cell tumors of bone. Radiology 134:441–446
14. Heelan RT, Watson RC, Smith J (1979) Computed tomography of lower extremity tumors. AJR 132:933–937
15. Helms CA, Cann CE, Brunelle FO, Gilula LA, Chafetz N, Genant HK (1981) Detection of bone-marrow metastases using quantitative computed tomography. Radiology 140:745–750
16. Hermann G, Rose JS (1979) Computed tomography in bone and soft tissue pathology of the extremities. J Comput Assist Tomogr 3:58–66
17. Hinderling T, Ruegsegger P, Anliker M, Dietschi C (1979) Computed tomography reconstruction from hollow projections: An application to in vivo evaluation of artificial hip joints. J Comput Assist Tomogr 3:52–57
18. Jend HH, Heller M, Schontag H, Schoettle H (1980) A computer tomographic method for the determination of tibial torsion. Rofo 133:22–25
19. Judet J, Judet H, Massare C (1979) Le scanner dans l'exploration des malpositions rotuliennes. Chirurgie 105:535–539
20. Kenney P, Gilula LA, Murphy WA (1981) The use of computed tomography to distinguish osteochondroma and chondrosarcoma. Radiology 139:129–137
21. Lange TA, Alter AJ (1980) Evaluation of complex acetabular fractures by computed tomography. Comput Assist Tomogr 4:849–852
22. Lange S, Weiss T, Gahl G, Golde G (1978) Knochendichtemessung mit dem Computertomographen. Rofo 129:66–69
23. Larsson S, Bergstrom M, Dahlqvist T, Israelsson A, Lagergren C (1978) A method for determining bone mineral content using fourier image reconstruction and dual source technique. J Comput Assist Tomogr 2:347–351
24. Lasda NA, Levinsohn EM, Yuan HA, Bunnell WP (1978) Computerized tomography in disorders of the hip. J Bone Joint Surg [Am] 60:1099–1102
25. Levinsohn EM (1979) Categorical course in CT. RE Buenger, ed, presented at RSNA, 809 (A) 2-2:2–14
26. Levinsohn EM, Bryan PJ (1979) Computed tomography in unilateral extremity swelling of unusual cause. J Comput Assist Tomogr 3:67–70
27. Levinshon EM, Bunnell WP, Yuan HA (1979) Computed tomography in the diagnosis of dislocations of the sternoclavicular joint. Clin Orthop 140:12–16
28. Lloyd TV, Paul DJ (1979) Erosion of the scapula by a benign lipoma: Computed tomography diagnosis. J Comput Assist Tomogr 3:679–680
29. Massare C (1980) Apport du scanner dans le diagnostic des desequilibres rotuliens. Rev Chir Orthop 4:233–237
30. Mayes GB, Wallace S, Bernardino ME (1981) Computed tomography of chondrosarcoma. CT 5(4):345–348
31. Naidich DP, Freedman MT, Bowerman JW, Siegelman SS (1978) Computerized tomography in the evaluation of the soft tissue component of bony lesions of the pelvis. Skeletal Radiol 3:144–148
32. Padovani J, Faure F, Devred P, Jacquemier M, Sarrat P (1979) Interet et indications de la tomodensitometrie dans le bilan des luxations congenitales de la hanche. Ann Radiol 22:188–193
33. Penkava RR (1980) Iliopsoas bursitis demonstrated by computed tomography. AJR 135:175–176
34. Peters JC, Coleman BG, Turner ML, Arger PH, Mulhern CBI, Dalinka MK, Allan DA, Schumacher HR (1980) CT evaluation of enlarged iliopsoas bursa. AJR 135:392–394
35. Revak CS, Gordan GS, Mazess RB, Wilson CR, Cann CE, Genani HK, Boyd DP, Gould RG, Kaufman L (1979) Proceedings of the international workshop on bone and soft tissue densitometry using computed tomography. San Francisco, California, 7–9 June 1979. J Comput Assist Tomogr. 3:847–862
36. Ram PC, Martinez S, Korobkin M, Breiman RS, Gallis HR, Harrelson JM (1981) CT detection of intraosseous gas: A new sign of osteomyelitis. AJR 137:721–723
37. Ruegsegger P, Anliker M, Dambacher M (1981) Quantification of trabecular bone with low dose computed tomography. J Comput Assist Thomogr 5:384–390
38. Sauser DD, Billimoria PE, Rouse GA, Mudge K (1980) CT evaluation of hip trauma. AJR 135:269–274
39. Shirkhoda A, Brashear R, Staab EV (1980) Computed tomography of acetabular fractures. Radiology 134:683–688
40. Stephenson TF (1980) Computerized tomography of soft tissue abnormalities. Comput Tomogr 4:181–188
41. Termote JL, Baert A, Crolla D, Palmers Y, Bulcke JA (1980) Computed tomography of the normal and pathologic muscular system. Radiology 137:439–444
42. Von Bazan B, Redlich UJ, Puhl W, Best S (1978) Das Os omovertebrale—neue Diagnostische Möglichkeit: die Axiale Computertomographie. Z Orthop 116:795–802

CHAPTER 7

Myopathies

J.A. BULCKE and P. DE MAEYER

The contribution of the radiologist to the investigation of muscle diseases has so far been rather limited, although some radiological and radioisotope procedures for examination of muscle have been available for many years [1–5]. Even though CT scanning is put to extensive use for the examination of almost every part of the body, only a few reports have described CT of the musculoskeletal system and myopathies [6–9].

In this chapter the application of CT scanning to the study of myopathies will be illustrated by five different cases of muscle disease. Each diagnosis was thoroughly verified during extensive investigation in hospital. Scans of the pelvic muscles, the thighs and the lower legs were selected for presentation in each case because they represent functional entities in which the most interesting radiological features of myopathy were found. The right and left side of the scans have to be read as in classical radiology.

Shown first (Figs. 7.1, 7.2) are two cases of an X-linked muscular dystrophy known as Becker's Disease, which is rather similar in clinical appearance to Duchenne's Disease but has a more benign clinical course [10]. The radiological appearance of each case can be considered pathognomonic and diagnostic for this disease. In Fig. 7.3 a case of polymyositis is shown. This autoimmune muscle disorder has been selected for presentation because it is a classical example of the many myopathies in which the earliest muscles to be affected are the proximal shoulder and pelvic girdle muscles, in contrast to the rarer distal myopathies, an example of which is illustrated in Fig. 7.4. The specific "vacuolar" radiological appearance of polymyositis is also pointed out. Spinal muscular atrophies or lower motor neuron diseases have a more diffuse atrophy pattern, as shown in Fig. 7.5, which can also be considered an example of the end stage of myopathy. The "ragged" appearance of the muscles in this disease seems to be a diagnostic feature of spinal muscular atrophy.

The term "atrophy" is used to describe muscle degeneration, and does not necessarily imply muscle hypotrophy or diminished muscle mass. One of the most striking features of myopathies revealed only by CT scanning is indeed that the process of muscle degeneration consists of a poorly understood [11] process of infiltration of the muscle by connective tissue while the original space within the fascia remains essentially the same, making transcutaneous appraisal of the degree of muscle atrophy almost impossible. Far-reaching destruction can remain hidden from the clinical observer: even extensive testing of muscle strength gives an unreliable impression of the degree of atrophy, and the same is certainly true for the clinical testing of muscle power. For example, the patient shown in Fig. 2 is still walking around without aid and only an experienced observer could make an adequate guess at the degree of muscle atrophy.

Not only has CT scanning greatly enhanced our ability to assess the extent of muscle destruction caused by myopathies and to obtain insight into the processes of muscle degeneration, but it also entails numerous clinical and other applications, such as follow-up of patients, selection of most suitable biopsy sites, evaluation of EMG data in the area of EMG potential sampling [12], follow-up of training results in athletes and obtainment of medicolegal proof of traumatic lesions which cannot otherwise be proved.

A description of the normal musculoskeletal system has been given elsewhere [13] and will not be repeated here.

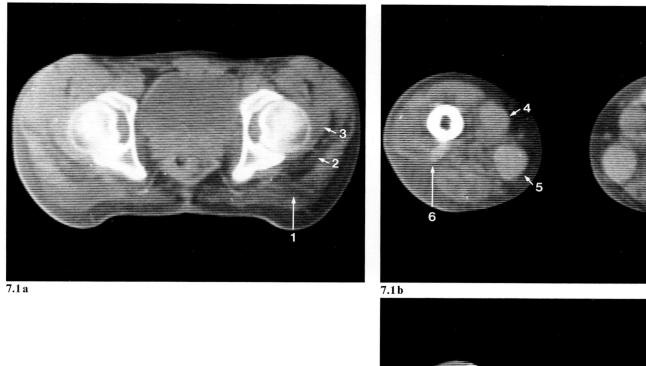

7.1a

7.1b

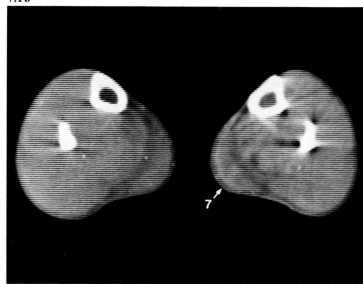

7.1c

Fig. 7.1 a–c. Becker's muscular dystrophy in a 25-year-old male.

a CT scan through the pelvic muscles approximately at the level of the middle of the inguinal ligament. Atrophy of the posterior pelvic muscles, starting with the gluteus maximus muscle (*1*) and progressing into the gluteus medius (*2*) is an early and very typical diagnostic feature. The gluteus minimus (*3*) is still well preserved.

b Thigh muscles 15 cm above the upper edge of the patella. Diffuse, moderate and symmetrical atrophy of all muscles can be seen, but with very typical selective preservation and (compensatory?) hyper-

trophy of the sartorius muscle (*4*) and particularly of the gracilis muscle (*5*). In this case the short head of the biceps femoris muscle (*6*) is also selectively spared. Earlier stages are characterized by hypertrophy of the semitendinosus muscle very similar to that of the gracilis muscle.

c Lower leg muscles 20 cm below the upper edge of the patella. The lower leg is clearly hypertrophic but the interior muscle mass of the medial head (*7*) of the gastrocnemius muscle has become infiltrated by fat tissue. This is a transitional stage between true hypertrophy and pseudohypertrophy and always starts at this site in this disease

185

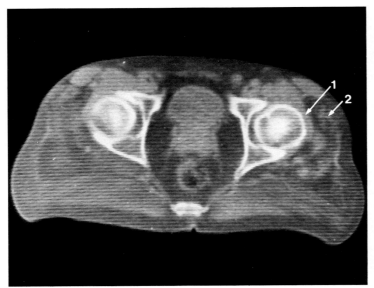

7.2a

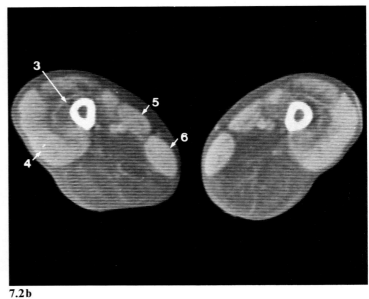

7.2b

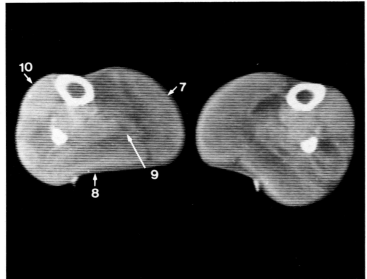

7.2c

Fig. 7.2a–c. Becker's muscular dystrophy in a 50-year-old male.

a CT scan through the pelvic muscles at the level of the middle of the inguinal ligament. The atrophy of the posterior pelvic muscles is very similar to that shown in Fig. 7.1, but has progressed further to include the gluteus minimus muscle (*1*) and the tensor fasciae latae muscle (*2*).

b Thigh muscles 15 cm above the upper edge of the patella. Here also the muscle atrophy has progressed further, and therefore the selectivity of the atrophy is much more pronounced. The hamstring muscles are almost completely infiltrated by low-density tissue, only fragments of the fasciae remaining visible. The quadriceps muscle is much better preserved, however, and it can clearly be seen that atrophy in this muscle progresses from the inner vastus intermedius muscle (*3*) towards the periphery, the vastus lateralis (*4*) being relatively spared. Here again the sartorius (*5*) and gracilis (*6*) muscles show their typical hypertrophic appearance.

c Lower leg muscles 20 cm below the upper edge of the patella. The lower legs are hypertrophic but the muscles show infiltration by low-density tissue in both the medial (*7*) and lateral (*8*) heads of the gastrocnemius muscle, and in the soleus muscle (*9*). The tibialis anterior muscle (*10*), is dense and hypertrophic. This is a typical image of pseudohypertrophy, the hypertrophy being made up of a mixture of fat and muscle tissue

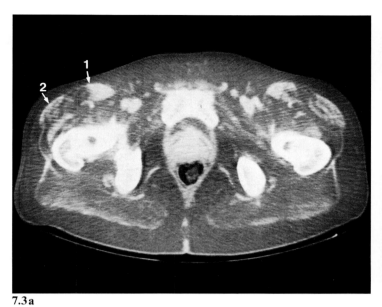

7.3a

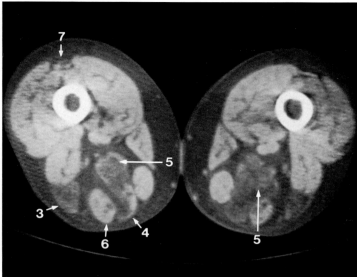

7.3b

7.3c

Fig. 7.3a–c. Polymyositis in a 40-year-old male.

a CT scan through the pelvic muscles halfway between the upper and lower edges of the pubic symphysis. Severe generalized atrophy is seen in all muscle groups. Only the fasciae of the muscles can still be observed, with residual muscle tissue of the sartorius (*1*) and tensor fasciae latae (*2*) muscles.

b Thigh muscles 15 cm above the upper edge of the patella. The muscles at this level are much better preserved, and severe atrophy is limited to symmetrical parts of the long head (*3*) of the biceps

femoris muscle, the semimembranosus muscle (*4*) and the adductor muscles (*5*). Milder and partial atrophy is present in the semitendinosus muscle (*6*). The other muscles, in particular the quadriceps, are better preserved, although the rectus femoris muscle (*7*) is selectively and severely atrophic on both sides.

c Lower leg muscles 20 cm below the upper edge of the patella. No specific atrophy of any particular muscle can be seen, but all muscles are diffusely infiltrated by lower-density tissue and have a vacuolar appearance, which can be considered diagnostic of polymyositis and is probably due to myo-oedema

187

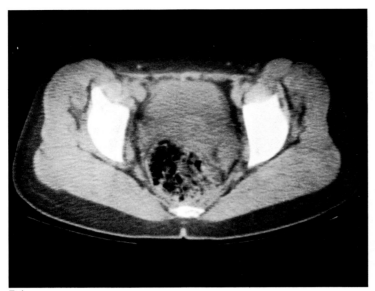

7.4a

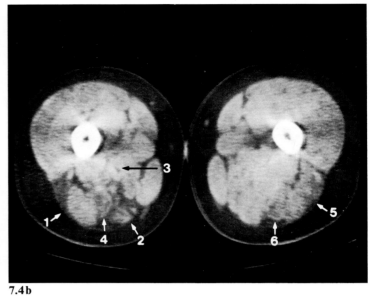

7.4b

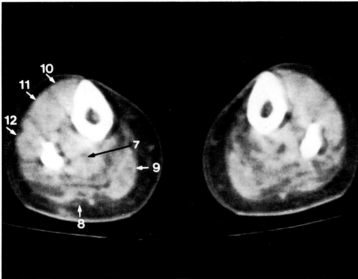

7.4c

Fig. 7.4a–c. Autosomal dominant distal muscular dystrophy in a 26-year-old female.

a CT scan through the pelvic muscles approximately at the level of the middle of the inguinal ligament. This scan can be considered normal. All muscle masses are normal in size and density.

b Thigh muscles 15 cm above the upper edge of the patella. Moderate atrophy of the hamstring muscles is seen on the left. More particularly, a triangular area of the long head of the biceps femoris muscle (*1*), the semimembranosus muscle (*2*) and the semitendinosus muscle

(*4*) are affected. Mild atrophy is also present in the adductor magnus muscle (*3*). On the right the atrophy is much less pronounced, but a decrease in density of the biceps femoris muscle (*5*) and probably also the semitendinosus muscle (*6*) can be seen.

c Lower leg muscles 20 cm below the upper edge of the patella. The soleus muscle (*7*) and the gastrocnemius muscle and its lateral head (*8*) are severely affected, the medial head of the gastrocnemius muscle somewhat less so. Better preserved are the anterior and lateral tibial muscles: tibialis anterior (*10*), extensor digitorum longus (*11*) and peroneus longus (*12*)

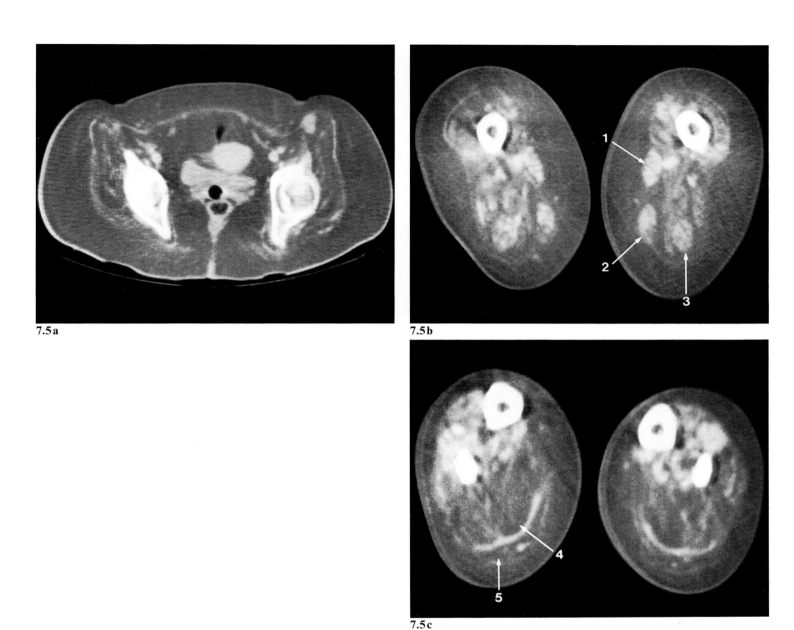

7.5a

7.5b

7.5c

Fig. 7.5a–c. Autosomal recessive spinal muscular atrophy (Kugelberg-Welander type) in a 32-year-old female.

a CT scan of the pelvic muscles halfway between the upper and lower edges of the pubic symphysis. Total disappearance of normal muscle tissue can be observed. Only fasciae, vascular and nervous structures can still be identified, together with a number of small islands of muscle tissue located within the previous muscle mass. Note that the total volume of the soft tissues has been preserved; the same is true in **b** and **c**.

b Thigh muscles 15 cm above the upper edge of the patella. Severe generalized atrophy of all muscles can be seen with a ragged appear-

ance, which can be considered typical for lower motor neuron diseases and is different from any other myopathy studied so far. The contour of the quadriceps muscle can still be seen, together with three better-preserved muscles: sartorius (*1*), gracilis (*2*) and (probably) semitendinosus (*3*).

c Lower leg muscles 20 cm below the upper edge of the patella. Total atrophy can be seen of both the soleus muscle (*4*) and the gastrocnemius muscle (*5*). The anterior tibial muscles are still visible but also demonstrate the ragged appearance of the thigh muscles

References

1. Di Chiro G, Nelson KB (1965) Soft tissue radiography of extremities in neuromuscular disease with histological correlations. Acta Radiol [Diagn] 3:65–68
2. Pálvölgyi R (1978) Roentgenological findings in muscular alterations of extremities. Radiologe 18:469–474
3. Pálvölgyi R (1979) Roentgenmorphological muscle changes in anterior horn cell lesions. Fortschr Röntgenstr 130:338–341
4. Siegel BA, Engel WK, Derrer EC (1975) 99mTc-diphosphate uptake in skeletal muscle: A quantitative index of acute damage. Neurology 25:1055–1058
5. Bellina CR, Bianchi R, Bombardieri S, Ferri C, Mariani G, Muratorio A, Rossi B (1978) Quantitative evaluation of 99m Tc-pyrophosphate muscle uptake in patients with inflammatory and non-inflammatory muscle diseases. J Nucl Med 22:89–96
6. O'Doherty DS, Schellinger D, Raptopoulos V (1977) Computed tomographic patterns of pseudohypertrophic muscular dystrophy: Preliminary results. J Comput Assist Tomogr 1:482–486
7. Häggmark T, Jansson E, Svane B (1978) Cross-sectional area of thigh muscle in man measured by computed tomography. Scand J Clin Lab Invest 38:355–360
8. Termote JL, Baert A, Crolla D, Palmers Y, Bulcke JA (1980) Computed tomography of the normal and pathological muscular system. Radiology 137:439–444
9. Bulcke JA, Crolla D, Termote JL, Baert A, Palmers Y, Van Den Bergh R (1981) Computed tomography of muscle. Muscle Nerve 4:67–72
10. Emery AEH, Skinner R (1976) Clinical studies in benign (Becker type) X-linked muscular dystrophy. Clin Genet 10:189–201
11. Duance VC, Stephens HR, Dunn M, Bailey AJ, Dubowitz V (1980) A role of collagen in the pathogenesis of muscular dystrophy? Nature 284:470–472
12. Bulcke JA, De Meirsman J, Termote JL (1979) The influence of skeletal muscle atrophy on needle electromyography. As demonstrated by computed tomography. EMG Clin Neurophysiol 19:269–279
13. Bulcke JA, Termote JL, Palmers Y, Crolla D (1979) Computed tomography of the human skeletal muscular system. Neuroradiology 17:127–136

Subject Index

Illustrated Computer Tomography

A Practical Guide to CT Interpretations

Editor: **S. Takahashi**
With the assistance of S. Sakuma, M. Kaneko
1983. 313 figures, partly colored. XII, 306 pages. ISBN 3-540-11432-7

Contents: Introduction. – Basic Aspects of Computed Tomography. – Atlas of Computed Tomography of the Normal Adult. – Clinical Application of Computed Tomography. – Radiotherapy Planning and Computed Tomography. – References. – Subject Index.

Here at last is the guide practitioners have been waiting for. Written by leading authorities in fields ranging from diagnostic radiology to neurosurgery and medical technology, it is the first to provide a comprehensive modern atlas of normal CT scans and their corresponding anatomical sections as a preliminary to CT imaging in clinical abnormalities. The book opens with a discussion of the basic aspects of computer tomography: its history and principles, apparatus, procedures, and image evaluation. Part 2 contains a complete atlas of axial transverse CT cross sections in the normal adult, complemented by antero-posterior and lateral X-ray views and anatomical diagrams for each CT image. This is designed to ficilitate understanding of the clinical applications of CT in the diagnosis and treatment of diseases of the brain, head and neck, trunk, and extremities described in Part 3. The book concludes with a consideration of the role of computer tomography in radiotherapy planning.
With the ever-increasing significance of computer tomography in today's medicine this book will prove indispensable for every physician seeking firm understanding of an important diagnostic tool.

J.A.L. Bulcke, A.L. Baert

Clinical and Radiological Aspects of Myopathies

CT Scanning – EMG – Radioisotopes
1982. 151 figures, 30 tables. XI, 187 pages. ISBN 3-540-11443-2

G. B. Bradač, R. Oberson

Angiography and Computed Tomography in Cerebro-Arterial Occlusive Diseases

With a Foreword by J.-M. Taveras
2nd, revised and expanded edition. 1983. 146 figures in 389 separate illustrations.
XII, 290 pages. ISBN 3-540-11453-X

H. Petterson, D.C.F. Harwood-Nash

CT and Myelography of the Spine and Cord

Techniques, Anatomy and Pathology in Children

In association with C.R. Fitz, S. Chuang
1982. 93 figures. XIII, 119 pages. ISBN 3-540-11322-2

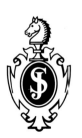

Springer-Verlag
Berlin
Heidelberg
New York
Tokyo

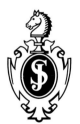